High-Yield™

Cell and Molecular Biology

THIRD EDITION

High-Yield™

Cell and Molecular Biology

THIRD EDITION

Ronald W. Dudek, PhD

Professor
Brody School of Medicine
East Carolina University
Department of Anatomy and Cell Biology
Greenville, North Carolina

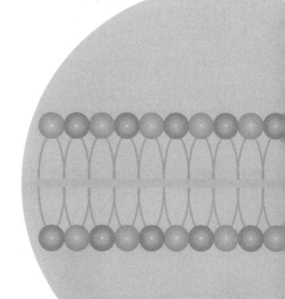

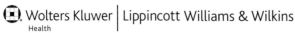
Wolters Kluwer | Lippincott Williams & Wilkins
Health

Philadelphia · Baltimore · New York · London
Buenos Aires · Hong Kong · Sydney · Tokyo

Acquisitions Editor: Crystal Taylor
Product Manager: Stacey Sebring
Vendor Manager: Alicia Jackson
Designer: Teresa Mallon
Compositor: Aptara, Inc.

Third Edition

Printed in China

First Edition, 1999
Second Edition, 2007

Library of Congress Cataloging-in-Publication Data

Dudek, Ronald W., 1950-
  High-yield cell and molecular biology / Ronald W. Dudek.—3rd ed.
       p. ; cm. — (High-yield)
  Cell and molecular biology
  Includes bibliographical references and index.
  ISBN 978-1-60913-573-7 (alk. paper)
  1. Molecular biology—Outlines, syllabi, etc.   2. Pathology—Outlines, syllabi, etc.   3. Cytology—Outlines, syllabi, etc.
I. Title.   II. Title: Cell and molecular biology.   III. Series: High-yield series.
  [DNLM: 1. Molecular Biology—Outlines.   2. Cell Biology—Outlines.   QU 18.2]
  QH506.D83 2012
  572.8—dc22
                                                                        2010038481

To purchase additional copies of this book, call our customer service department at **(800) 638-3030** or fax orders to **(301) 223-2320.** International customers should call **(301) 223-2300.**

Visit Lippincott Williams & Wilkins on the Internet: http://www.lww.com. Lippincott Williams & Wilkins customer service representatives are available from 8:30 am to 6:00 pm, EST.

This book is dedicated to my good friend Ronald Cicinelli, who is now a retired vice-president of The Chase Bank. In our 40 years of friendship, I have witnessed his dedication to family and friends. Ron brings a unique combination of strength and kindness to every personal interaction. I have been honored to know him for all these years. His life has been and continues to be, a "high-yield" life.

This book is also dedicated to my godson Alec Ronald Walker, born April 28, 2005. Alec joins a remarkable and loving family of parents Tim and Laura, sister Gabriella, and brother Brandson. Alec will certainly be given all the guidance necessary for a successful life, which will give me great joy to witness. My admonishment to my dear godson is to remember: "To whom much is given, much is expected."

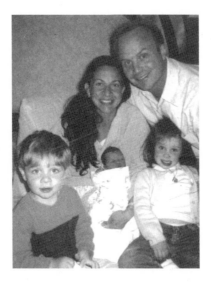

Preface

The impact of molecular biology today and in the future cannot be underestimated. Gene therapy and cloning of sheep are explained and discussed in the daily newspapers.

The clinical and etiological aspects of diseases are now being explained at the molecular biology level. Drugs are being designed right now by various pharmaceutical companies to impact molecular biological processes in the treatment of disease (cancer, obesity, etc.). Molecular biology will be increasingly represented on the USMLE Step 1. One of my main concerns in writing this book was NOT to write a review of basic molecular biology but to write a book that addressed molecular biology from a clinical perspective that would be useful and necessary for our future physicians. I was greatly assisted in this matter by two medical students who took an unsolicited interest in "High Yield Cell and Molecular Biology" third edition because they appreciated the growing importance of molecular biology for the future physician. In this regard, I would like to acknowledge the significant contribution of Mr. Jonah Cohen, a third–fourth-year student at the Brown Medical School and published cancer researcher in NF-κB signal transduction, and Mr. Fateh Bazerbachi, a third-year student at Damascus University School of Medicine (Syria). Jonah Cohen was especially helpful in limiting the scope of material to hone in on the most clinically relevant issues and eliminating some far-reaching material that was included in the second edition. Fateh Bazerbachi was especially helpful in identifying new information and clarifying some difficult areas to understand. I found their assistance to be very helpful and it should benefit all my readers.

How will medical schools teach the clinical relevance of molecular biology to our future physicians? Medical school curricula are already filled with needed and relevant "traditional" courses. Where will the time needed to teach a molecular biology course be found? I suspect what will happen is that many of the "traditional" courses will extend their discussion of various topics down to the molecular biology level. This approach will work, but it will in effect make molecular biology somewhat disjointed. The student will learn some molecular biology in a biochemistry course, some in a microbiology course, and some in a histology course, etc. The problem this presents for students reviewing for USMLE Step 1 is that molecular biology information will be scattered among various course notes.

The solution: High Yield Cell and Molecular Biology, third edition. In this third edition, I have consolidated the important clinical issues related to molecular biology that are obvious "grist-for-the-mill" for USMLE Step 1 questions and included many of the insightful suggestions of my readers and reviewers. It is my feeling that "High Yield Cell and Molecular Biology" will be of tremendous benefit to any serious review for USMLE Step 1. Please send your feedback, comments, and suggestions to me at dudekr@ecu.edu for inclusion into the next edition.

Ronald W. Dudek, PhD

Contents

Preface vii
Abbreviations xiii

1 Chromosomal DNA 1

    I. The Biochemistry of Nucleic Acids 1
    II. Levels of DNA Packaging 2
    III. Centromere 4
    IV. Heterochromatin 4
    V. Euchromatin 4
    VI. Studying Human Chromosomes 4
    VII. Staining of Chromosomes 5
    VIII. Chromosome Morphology 6
    IX. DNA Melting Curve 7

2 Chromosome Replication 9

    I. General Features 9
    II. The Chromosome Replication Process .9
    III. DNA Topoisomerases 11
    IV. The Telomere 12
    V. DNA Damage 12
    VI. DNA Repair 13
    VII. Clinical Considerations 14
    VIII. Summary of Chromosome Replication Machinery 16

3 Meiosis and Genetic Recombination 17

    I. Meiosis 17
    II. Genetic Recombination 19

4 The Human Nuclear Genome 22

    I. General Features 22
    II. Protein-Coding Genes 23
    III. RNA-Coding Genes 24
    IV. Epigenetic Control. 25
    V. Noncoding DNA 25

5 The Human Mitochondrial Genome 29

   I.   General Features 29
   II. The 13 Protein-Coding Genes 29
   III. The 24 RNA-Coding Genes 29
   IV. Other Mitochondrial Proteins 31
   V. Mitochondrial Diseases 31

6 Protein Synthesis 33

   I.   General Features 33
   II. Transcription 33
   III. Processing the RNA Transcript into mRNA 34
   IV. Translation 35
   V. Clinical Considerations 37

7 Control of Gene Expression 39

   I.   General Features 39
   II. Mechanism of Gene Expression 39
   III. The Structure of DNA-Binding Proteins. 41
   IV. Other Mechanisms of Gene Expression 44
   V. The *Lac* Operon 46
   VI. The *trp* Operon 47

8 Mutations of the DNA Sequence 49

   I.   General Features 49
   II. Silent (Synonymous) Mutations. 49
   III. Non-Silent (Nonsynonymous) Mutations 50
   IV. Loss of Function and Gain of Function Mutations 55
   V. Other Types of Polymorphisms 56

9 Proto-Oncogenes, Oncogenes, and Tumor-Suppressor Genes 58

   I.   Proto-Oncogenes and Oncogenes 58
   II. Tumor-Suppressor Genes 60
   III. Hereditary Cancer Syndromes 62

10 The Cell Cycle 66

   I.   Mitosis 66
   II. Control of the Cell Cycle 68

11 Molecular Biology of Cancer 71

   I.   The Development of Cancer (Oncogenesis) 71
   II. The Progression of Cancer 72
   III. Signal Transduction Pathways 73

12 Cell Biology of the Immune System 77

    I. Neutrophils (Polys, Segs, or PMNs) 77
    II. Eosinophils 78
    III. Basophils 78
    IV. Mast Cells 78
    V. Monocytes 79
    VI. Macrophages (Histiocytes; Antigen-Presenting Cells) 80
    VII. Natural Killer CD16$^+$ Cell 81
    VIII. B Lymphocyte 81
    IX. T Lymphocyte 83
    X. Immune Response to Exogenous Protein Antigens 85
    XI. Immune Response to Endogenous Antigens (Intracellular Virus or Bacteria) 86
    XII. Cytokines 87

13 Molecular Biology of the Immune System 89

    I. Clonal Selection Theory 89
    II. The B Lymphocyte (B Cell) 89
    III. The T Lymphocyte (T Cell) 93
    IV. Clinical Considerations 95
    V. Disorders of Phagocytic Function 96
    VI. Systemic Autoimmune Disorders 97
    VII. Organ-Specific Autoimmune Disorders 97

14 Molecular Biology Techniques 100

    I. Action of Restriction Enzymes 101
    II. Electrophoresis 103
    III. The Enzymatic Method of DNA Sequencing 105
    IV. Southern Blotting and Prenatal Testing for Sickle Cell Anemia 107
    V. Isolating a Human Gene by DNA Cloning 109
    VI. Construction of cDNA Library 111
    VII. Polymerase Chain Reaction 113
    VIII. Producing a Protein from a Cloned Gene 115
    IX. Site-Directed Mutagenesis and Knockout Animals 117
    X. Northern Blot (mRNA) 119
    XI. Western Blot (Protein) 121
    XII. Human Immunodeficiency Virus (HIV) Structure 123
    XIII. Ligase Chain Reaction (LCR) 125
    XIV. Flow Cytometry 127

15 Identification of Human Disease Genes 129

    I. General Features 129
    II. Identification of a Human Disease Gene Through a Chromosome Abnormality 129
    III. Identification of a Human Disease Gene Through Pure Transcript Mapping 130
    IV. Identification of a Human Disease Gene Through Large Scale DNA Sequencing 131
    V. Identification of a Human Disease Gene Through Comparison of Human and Mouse Maps 132

16 **Gene Therapy** 133

    I. Gene Therapy 133
    II. Ex Vivo and In Vivo Gene Therapy 134
    III. Integration into Host Cell Chromosomes or as Episomes 134
    IV. Viral Vectors Used in Gene Therapy 134
    V. Nonviral Vectors Used in Gene Therapy 135

Appendix 1: The Genetic Code 137
Appendix 2: Amino Acids 138
Appendix 3: Chromosomal Locations of Human Genetic Diseases 139
Figure Credits 145
Index 147

Abbreviations

5-HT	**5**-**h**ydroxy**t**ryptamine
ABC	**A**TP-**b**inding **c**assette
ABL	**Ab**elson murine **l**eukemia
abl/bcr	**Ab**elson murine **l**eukemia viral gene/**b**reakpoint **c**luster **r**egion oncogene
abl	**Ab**elson mouse **l**eukemia
AC	**a**denylate **c**yclase
ACTH	**a**dreno**c**ortico**t**ropin **h**ormone
ADA	**a**denosine **dea**minase
ADH	**a**nti**di**uretic **h**ormone or vasopressin
AMPA	α-**am**ino-3-hydroxy-5-methyl-4-isoxazole **p**ropionic **a**cid
ANP	**a**trial **n**atriuretic **p**eptide
anti-MuSK	anti-**mu**scle **s**pecific receptor tyrosine **k**inase
AP1	**a**ctivator **p**rotein -1
Apaf-1	**a**poptotic **p**eptidase **a**ctivating **f**actor
APC	familial **a**denomatous **p**olyposis **c**oli
AT_1	**a**ngio**t**ensin
ATM	**a**taxia **t**elangiectasia **m**utated
ATR	**a**taxia **t**elangiectasia and **R**AD3- related
B_1 and B_2	**b**radykinin$_{1,2}$ receptors
BACs	**b**acterial **a**rtificial **c**hromosomes based on the F-factor plasmids
BASC	BRCA1-**a**ssociated genome **s**urveillance **c**omplex
BAT	**b**iliary **a**cid **t**ransporter
Bcl-2	**B**-cell **C**LL/**l**ymphoma 2
BCR	**b**reakpoint **c**luster **r**egion
BK_{Ca}	large (**b**ig) conductance **Ca**$^{2+}$-activated **K**$^+$ channel protein
BLM	**Bl**oo**m**
BOR	**b**ranchio-**o**to-**r**enal
BRCA	**br**east **ca**ncer
Btk	**B**ruton **t**yrosine **k**inase
C bands	**c**onstitutive heterochromatin bands
C/EBP	**C**CAAT/**e**nhancer **b**inding **p**rotein
CaM-kinase	**Ca**$^{++}$/cal**m**odulin-dependent protein kinase
CAP	**c**atabolite **a**ctivator **p**rotein
CCK	**c**hole**c**ysto**k**inin
CCP	**c**itrulline **c**ontaining **p**roteins
CD 40	**c**luster of **d**ifferentiation 40
CD40LG	**c**luster of **d**ifferentiation 40 **lig**and
CENP	**cen**tromeric **p**roteins
CF	**c**ystic **f**ibrosis
CGH	**c**omparative **g**enome **h**ybridization
Chk	**ch**eckpoint **k**inase
COMT	**c**atechol-**O**-**m**ethyl**t**ransferase
cosmid	**co**hesive **s**ticky ends of the bacteriophage λ inserted into a plas**mid**
COX	**c**ycl**oox**ygenase I and II
CRE	**c**AMP **r**esponse **e**lement
CREB	**c**AMP **r**esponse **e**lement **b**inding protein
CTP	**c**itrate **t**ransport **p**rotein
CURL	**c**ompartment for **u**ncoupling of **r**eceptor and **l**igand
CYBB	**cy**tochrome **b**-245 **b**eta polypeptide; also called gp91
D1, D2	**d**opamine 1,2
DAG	**di**a**c**yl**g**lycerol
DCC	**d**eleted in **c**olon **c**arcinoma

DDB2	damage-specific DNA binding gene 2
DGCR	DiGeorge chromosomal region
DPE	downstream promoter element
DSCR	Down syndrome critical region
E2F	elongation factor 2
EBV	Epstein Barr virus
EGF	epidermal growth factor
EGFR	epidermal growth factor receptor
ELN	elastin
env	envelope
erb	erythroblastosis
ERCC3	excision repair cross-complementing (rodent gene)
ERG	erythroblastosis virus E26 oncogene like (avian)
ERV	endogenous retroviral
EYA1	eyes absent gene 1
Fab	fragment; antigen binding
F-actin	filamentous actin
Fas	faint sausage
FAT	fatty acid transporter
F_C	fragment; crystallizable
fes	feline sarcoma
FGF	fibroblast growth factor
FISH	fluorescence in situ hybridization
FMR 1	fragile X mental retardation 1
Fos	Finkel-Biskes-Jinkins osteogenic sarcoma
FSH	follicle-stimulating hormone
FUS	fusion gene
G	trimeric GTP-binding proteins
G_0, G_1, G_2	gap zero, one, two
$GABA_A$	gamma-aminobutyric acid$_A$
GABRA 1	α1 subunit of the gamma-aminobutyric acid receptor subtype A 1
GAD_{65}	glutamic acid decarboxylase 65
gag	group specific antigens
G-CSF	granulocyte colony stimulating factor
GLUT1-5	glucose transporters 1-5
GM-CSF	granulocyte-monocyte colony stimulating factor
GpIb	platelet glycoprotein Ib
GRE	glucocorticoid response element
H_1, H_2	histamine$_{1,2}$
H2A, H2B, H3, H4	histone proteins
Ha-ras	Harvey mouse sarcoma-ras
HDV	human delta virus
HIV-1	human immunodeficiency virus-1
HLA	human leucocyte antigen
HLA-DRB1	major histocompatibility complex or human leukocyte antigen, class II, DR beta 1
HLH	helix-loop-helix
HMRE	heavy metal response element
Hsp	heat shock protein
HSRE	heat shock response element
IAP	inhibitor of apoptosis
IGH	immunoglobulin H
IKBKG	inhibitor of kappa light polypeptide gene enhancer in B cells, kinase gamma
IK_{Ca}	intermediate conductance Ca^{2+}-activated K$^+$ channel protein
IKK- gamma	I kappa B kinase gamma chain
IL-2	interleukin-2
Inr	initiator sequence
IP_3	inositol triphosphate
IRE	interferon-γ response element
ISP42	import site protein 42
ITGB2	integrin beta 2
K_A	transient outward rectifier voltage-gated K$^+$
K_{AA}	arachidonic acid modulated metabolically-gated K$^+$
K_{ACh}	acetylcholine-activated metabolically-gated K$^+$
K_{ATP}	ATP-sensitive metabolically-gated K$^+$
Kb	kilobase; a thousand (10^3) bases
K_{IR}	inward rectifier voltage-gated K$^+$
Ki-ras	Kirsten mouse sarcoma-ras
K_V	delayed rectifier voltage-gated K$^+$

lac operon	**lac**tose operon
LDL	**l**ow **d**ensity **l**ipoprotein
LH	**l**uteinizing **h**ormone
LIMK1	**l**in-11 **is**l-1 **mec**3 **k**inase 1
lin-4	abnormal cell **lin**eage-**4**
LINE	**l**ong **i**nterspersed **n**uclear **e**lement
LTB$_4$, LTC$_4$, LTD$_4$	**l**euko**t**riene B$_4$, C$_4$, D$_4$
LTR	**l**ong **t**erminal **r**epeat transposons
L-type Ca^{2+}	**l**ong-lasting **Ca^{2+}**
mACh	**m**uscarinic **a**cetyl**ch**oline
MaLR	**ma**mma**l**ian **r**etrotransposon-like
MAP	**m**itogen-**a**ctivated **p**rotein
Mb	**m**egabase; a million (10^6) bases
M-CSFR	**m**acrophage **c**olony-**s**timulating **f**actor **r**eceptor
Mdc1	**m**ediator of DNA **d**amage **c**heckpoint protein-**1**
MDM	**m**urine **d**ouble-**m**inute
MDR	**m**ulti**d**rug **r**esistance
Mep-1	**me**thionine amino **p**eptidase-**1**
mGlu	**m**etabotropic **glu**tamate receptor
MHC	**m**ajor **h**istocompatibility **c**omplex
miRNA	**mi**cro **r**ibo**n**ucleic **a**cid
MJD	**M**achado-**J**oseph **d**isease; SCA3
MLH	**m**utant **L** **h**omologue gene
MLL	**m**yeloid/**l**ymphoid or mixed-lineage **l**eukemia (trithorax homolog, Drosophila)
MOAT	**m**ultispecific **o**rgan **a**nion **t**ransporter
MSH	**m**utant **S** **h**omologue gene
MTOC	**m**icro**t**ubular **o**rganizing **c**enter
myb	**m**y**el**o**b**lastosis
myc	**m**y**el**o**c**ytosis virus gene
MyoD	**m**y**o**genic **d**ifferentiation 1 protein
nACh	**n**icotinic **a**cetyl**ch**oline receptor
NAD	**n**icotinamide **a**denine **d**inucleotide
NADH	**n**icotinamide **a**denine **d**inucleotide reduced form
NBT test	**n**itro**b**lue **t**etrazolium test
NEMO	**N**F-kappa B **e**ssential **mo**difier
NF	**n**uclear **f**actor
NF-1	**n**euro**f**ibromatosis
NFAT	**n**uclear **f**actor of **a**ctivated **T**-cells
NGF	**n**erve **g**rowth **f**actor
NMDA	**N**-**m**ethyl-**D**-**a**spartate
N-myc	**n**euroblastoma **m**y**e**lo**c**ytosis
N-ras	**n**euroblastoma **ras**
Nsd1	**n**uclear receptor-binding **S**ET-**d**omain **1**
NTRK	**n**eurotrophic **t**yrosine **k**inase **r**eceptor
OCT-1	**oct**anucleotide binding protein-**1**
p arm	**p**etite or short **arm** of a chromosome
P$_1$, P$_{2Y}$	**p**urinergic$_{1,2Y}$
P$_{2X}$	**p**urinergic$_{2X}$
PACs	**P**1 **a**rtificial **c**hromosomes based on the P1 bacteriophage
Pax3	**pa**ired bo**x** **3**
PBX1	**p**re-**B**-cell leukemia transcription factor **1**
PDGF	**p**latelet-**d**erived **g**rowth **f**actor
PHOX	**ph**agocyte NADPH **ox**idase
PIP$_2$	**p**hosphatidyl**i**nositol bi**p**hosphate
Pit-1	**pit**uitary specific factor-**1**
PKA	**p**rotein **k**inase **A**, which is a cAMP-dependent protein kinase
PKG	**p**rotein **k**inase **G**; a cGMP-dependent protein kinase
PL$_C$	**p**hospho**l**ipase **C**
PML	**p**ro**m**y**el**ocyte
*pml/rar*α	**p**ro**m**y**el**ocyte/**r**etinoic **a**cid **r**eceptor α
PMS	**p**ost **m**eiotic **s**egregation gene
Pol	**pol**ymerase
PRE	**p**horbol ester **r**esponse **e**lement
pro	**pro**tease
PTH	**pa**ra**t**hyroid **h**ormone
q arm	**q**ueue or long **arm** of a chromosome
Q bands	fluorochrome **q**uinacrine positive **bands**
R bands	Giemsa negative; light bands; **r**everse **bands**

RAG1	recombination activating gene-1
RARα	retinoic acid receptor α gene
ras gene	rat sarcoma gene
Rb	retinoblastoma
RISC	ribonucleic acid induced silencing complex
S phase	synthesis phase
SCA3/MJD	spinocerebellar ataxia/Machado-Joseph disease gene
SCID	severe combined immune deficiency
SCIDA	severe combined immune deficiency athabascan
SF-1	steroidogenic factor-1
SH2D1A	SH$_2$ domain protein 1A
SH$_2$-domain	sequence homology proteins
SINE	short interspersed nuclear element
siRNA	small interfering ribonucleic acid
sis	simian sarcoma
SK$_{Ca}$	small conductance Ca^{2+}-activated K$^+$
SLAM	signaling lymphocyte activation molecule
snoRNA	small nucleolar ribonucleic acid
snRNA	small nuclear ribonucleic acid
snRNP	small nuclear ribonucleoprotein particles
Sos	son-of-sevenless
SRA-1 RNA	steroid receptor activator 1 ribonucleic acid
Src	sarcoma
SRE	serum growth factor response element
SSB	single strand binding protein
SSR	simple sequence repeat
Stat-1	signal transduction and activation of transcription factor-1
T3,T4	thyroid hormone
TBP	TATA-binding protein
TCOF1	Treacher Collins Franceschetti 1
TDP	thymidine 5'-diphosphate
TFII	general transcription factors for RNA polymerase II)
TGFβ	transforming growth factor β receptor
TI	transcription initiation
TNF	tumor necrosis factor
TopBP1	topoisomerase binding protein 1
TPM3	tropomyosin 3
trp operon	tryptophan operon
TSH	thyroid stimulating hormone
T-type Ca^{2+}	transient Ca^{2+}
TXA$_2$	thromboxane A$_2$
UTR	untranslated region
uvrABC	UV radiation ATP-binding cassette
V$_1$,V$_2$	vasopressin$_{1,2}$ receptors
VCFS	velocardiofacial syndrome
VEGF	vascular endothelial growth factor
VHL	von Hippel-Lindau
VIP	vasoactive intestinal polypeptide
VS	Varkud satellite
WAGR	Wilms tumor, aniridia, genitourinary abnormalities, and mental retardation
WT1	Wilms tumor gene
Xce	X-controlling element
Xic	X-inactivation center
XIST	X inactive specific transcripts
XLA	X-linked Infantile agammaglobulinemia (Bruton)
XLP	X-linked lymphoproliferative Disease
XPV	xeroderma pigmentosum variant gene
YACs	yeast artificial chromosomes

Chapter 1

Chromosomal DNA

① **The Biochemistry of Nucleic Acids (Figure 1-1).** A nucleoside consists of a nitrogenous base and a sugar. A **nucleotide** consists of a nitrogenous base, a sugar, and a phosphate group. DNA and RNA consist of a chain of nucleotides, which are composed of the following components:

A. NITROGENOUS BASES
  1. Purines
    a. Adenine (A)
    b. Guanine (G)
  2. Pyrimidines
    a. Thymine (T)
    b. Cytosine (C)
    c. Uracil (U) which is found in RNA

B. SUGARS
  1. Deoxyribose
  2. Ribose which is found in RNA

C. PHOSPHATE (PO_4^{3-})

A

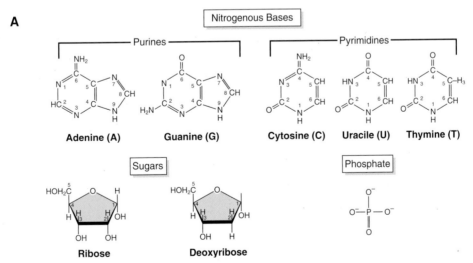

● **Figure 1-1 (A)** Structure of the biochemical components of DNA and RNA (purines, pyrimidines, sugars, and phosphate). (*continued*)

B

● **Figure 1-1** (*Continued*) **(B)** Diagram of a DNA polynucleotide chain. The biochemical components (purines, pyrimidines, sugar, and phosphate) form a polynucleotide chain through a 3′,5′-phosphodiester bond. If a piece of DNA contains 20% thymine, how much guanine does the piece of DNA contain? If the piece of DNA contains 20% thymine, then the piece of DNA will contain 20% adenine which equals 40% (thymine and adenine). The remaining 60% will consist of cytosine and guanine which are paired. Consequently, the piece of DNA will contain 30% guanine. A good mnemonic to remember which nitrogenous bases are purines is ***Pure As Gold*** (**A**denine and **G**uanine are ***Pur***ines).

Ⅱ Levels of DNA Packaging (Figure 1-2)

A. DOUBLE HELIX DNA

1.   The DNA molecule is two complementary polynucleotide chains (or DNA strands) arranged as a double helix which are held together by **hydrogen bonding** between laterally opposed base pairs (bps).

2.   DNA can adopt different helical structures which include: **A-DNA** and **B-DNA** which are right-handed helices with 11 and 10 bps per turn, respectively, and **Z-DNA** which is a left-handed helix with 12 bps per turn.

3.   In humans, most of the DNA is in the B-DNA form under physiological conditions.

B. NUCLEOSOME (Figure 1-2)

1. The most fundamental unit of DNA packaging is the **nucleosome**. A nucleosome consists of a **histone protein octamer** (two each of **H2A, H2B, H3, and H4 histone proteins**) around which 146 bps of DNA is coiled in 1.75 turns.

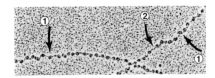

● Figure 1-2 Nucleosome.

2. The nucleosomes are connected by spacer DNA, which results in 10-nm diameter chromatin fiber that resembles a **"beads on a string"** appearance by electron microscopy. Figure 1-2 shows an electron micrograph of DNA that was isolated and subjected to treatments to unfold DNA into a 10-nm diameter chromatin fiber. The globular structure ("bead"; arrow 1) is the nucleosome. The linear structure ("string"; arrow 2) is spacer DNA.

3. The 10-nm diameter chromatin fiber is the first DNA structure that an endonuclease attacks in an apoptotic cell.

4. Histones are small proteins containing a high proportion of **lysine** and **arginine** that impart a positive charge to the proteins that enhances its binding to negatively charged DNA.

5. **Histone acetylation** reduces the affinity between histones and DNA. An increased acetylation of histone proteins will make a DNA segment more likely to be transcribed into RNA and hence any genes in that DNA segment will be expressed (i.e., ↑ **acetylation of histones = expressed genes**).

6. **Histone methylation** of lysine and arginine by **methyltransferases** also occurs.

C. 30-NM CHROMATIN FIBER

1. The 10-nm nucleosome fiber is joined by **H1 histone protein** to form a **30-nm chromatin fiber**.

2. During interphase of mitosis, chromosomes exist as 30-nm chromatin fibers organized in a **primary loop pattern** called **extended chromatin** (~300-nm diameter). The extended chromatin can also be organized in a **secondary loop pattern** as seen in condensed metaphase chromosomes. (*Note*: when the general term "chromatin" is used, it refers specifically to the 30-nm chromatin fiber organized as extended chromatin).

D. COMPACTION (Figure 1-3).

During metaphase of mitosis, chromosomes can become highly compacted. For example, human chromosome 1 contains about 260,000,000 bps. The distance between each base pair is 0.34 nm. So that the physical length of the DNA comprising chromosome 1 is 88,000,000 nm or 88,000 μm (260,000,000 × 0.34 nm = 88,000,000 nm). During metaphase, all the chromosomes condense such that the physical length of chromosome 1 is about 10 μm. Consequently, the 88,000 μm of DNA comprising chromosome 1 is reduced to 10 μm, resulting in a 8800-fold compaction. Figure 1-3 shows double helix DNA of chromosome 1 that is unraveled and stretched out measuring 88,000 μm in length. When chromosome 1 condenses as occurs during mitosis, the length is reduced to 10 μm. This is a 8800-fold compaction.

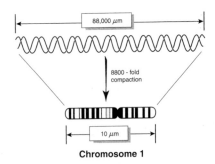

● Figure 1-3 Chromosome Compaction.

III Centromere

A. A centromere is a specialized nucleotide DNA sequence that binds to the **mitotic spindle during cell division.**

B. A major component of centromeric DNA is **α-satellite DNA** which consists of 171-bp repeat unit. **β-satellite DNA** (a 68-bp repeat unit) and **satellite 1 DNA** (25–48-bp repeat unit) are also components of centromeric DNA.

C. A centromere is also associated with a number of centromeric proteins, which include **CENP-A, CENP-B, CENP-C, and CENP-G.**

D. All chromosomes have a **single centromere** which is observed microscopically as a **primary constriction** and which is the region where sister chromatids are joined.

E. During prometaphase, a pair of protein complexes called **kinetochores** forms at the centromere where one kinetochore is attached to each sister chromatid.

F. Microtubules produced by the **centrosome** of the cell attached to the kinetochore (called **kinetochore microtubules**) and pull the two sister chromatids toward opposite poles of the mitotic cell.

IV Heterochromatin (Figure 1-4)

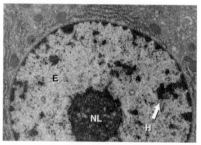

● Figure 1-4 Heterochromatin and Euchromatin.

A. Heterochromatin is **condensed chromatin** and comprises ~10% of the total chromatin.

B. Heterochromatin is **transcriptionally inactive** and is **electron dense** (i.e., very black) in electron micrographs.

C. An example of heterochromatin is the **Barr body** which is found in female cells and represents the inactive X chromosome.

D. **Constitutive heterochromatin** is always condensed (i.e., transcriptionally inactive) and consists of repetitive DNA found near the centromere and other regions.

E. **Facultative heterochromatin** can be either condensed (i.e., transcriptionally inactive) or dispersed (i.e., transcriptionally active).

F. The electron micrograph in Figure 1-4 shows a nucleus containing predominately euchromatin (E), peripherally located heterochromatin (H), and a centrally located nucleolus (NL).

V Euchromatin (Figure 1-4)

A. **EUCHROMATIN** is dispersed chromatin and comprises ~90% of the total chromatin.

B. Ten percent of euchromatin is **transcriptionally active** and 80% is **transcriptionally inactive.**

C. When chromatin is transcriptionally active, there is **weak binding to the H1 histone protein** and acetylation of the H2A, H2B, H3, and H4 histone proteins occurs.

VI Studying Human Chromosomes (Figure 1-5)

A. **MITOTIC CHROMOSOMES** are fairly easy to study because they can be observed in any cell undergoing mitosis.

B. **MEIOTIC CHROMOSOMES** are much more difficult to study because they can be observed only in ovarian or testicular samples. In the female, meiosis is especially difficult because meiosis occurs during fetal development. In the male, meiotic chromosomes can be studied only in a testicular biopsy of an adult male.

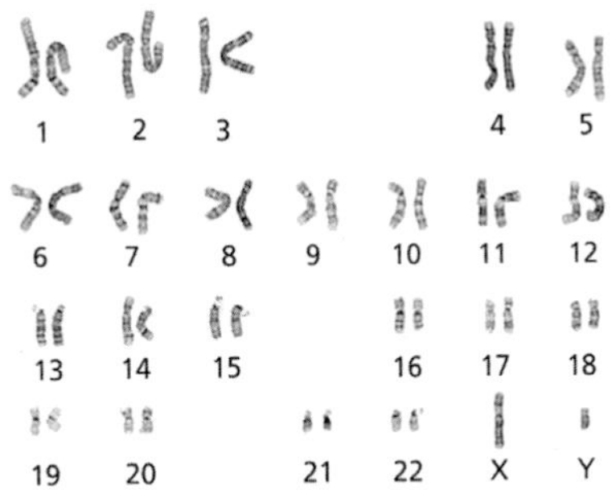

• Figure 1-5 Human Karyotype.

C. Blood is the most convenient source of human cells for **karyotype analysis**. Blood cells are cultured and a mitogen is added to the culture media to stimulate the **mitosis** of lymphocytes. Subsequently, **colchicine** is added to the media which arrests the lymphocytes in **metaphase**. It is often preferable to use **prometaphase** chromosomes because they are less condensed and therefore show more detail. The lymphocytes are then concentrated and treated with a hypotonic solution to lyse the lymphocytes and aid in spreading the chromosomes. The cell preparation is then spread on a microscope slide, fixed, and stained by a variety of methods (see section VII: Staining of Chromosomes). The separated metaphase chromosomes are then identified and photographed. The photos of all the chromosomes are then cut out and arranged in a standard pattern called the **karyotype**. Figure 1-5 shows the G-banding pattern of metaphase chromosomes arranged in a karyotype.

VII ## Staining of Chromosomes. Metaphase or prometaphase chromosomes are prepared for karyotype analysis (see section VI: Studying Human Chromosomes).

A. **CHROMOSOME BANDING.** The chromosome-banding technique is based on denaturation and/or enzymatic digestion of DNA followed by incorporation of a DNA-binding dye. This results in chromosomes staining as a series of dark and light bands.
   1. **G Banding**
      a. G banding uses the **Giemsa dye** and is now the standard analytical method in cytogenetics.
      b. Giemsa staining produces a unique pattern of **dark bands (Giemsa positive; G bands)** which consist of heterochromatin, replicate in the late S phase, are rich in A-T bases, and contain few genes.
      c. Giemsa staining also produces a unique pattern of **light bands (Giemsa negative; R bands)** which consist of euchromatin, replicate in the early S phase, rich in G–C bases, and contain many genes.
   2. **R Banding**
      a. R banding uses the Giemsa dye (as above) to visualize **light bands (Giemsa negative; R bands)** which are essentially the reverse of the G-banding pattern.
      b. R banding can also be visualized by G–C specific dyes (e.g., chromomycin A_3, oligomycin, or mithramycin).
   3. **Q Banding.** Q banding uses the fluorochrome quinacrine (binds preferentially to A–T bases) to visualize **Q bands** which are essentially the same as G bands.
   4. **T Banding.** T banding uses severe heat denaturation prior to Giemsa staining or a combination of dyes and fluorochromes to visualize **T bands** which are a subset of R bands located at the telomeres.
   5. **C Banding.** C banding uses barium hydroxide denaturation prior to Giemsa staining to visualize **C bands** which are constitutive heterochromatin located mainly at the centromere.

B. FLUORESCENCE IN SITU HYBRIDIZATION (FISH)

1. The FISH technique is based on the ability of single-stranded DNA (i.e., a DNA probe) to hybridize (bind or anneal) to its complementary target sequence on a unique DNA sequence that one is interested in localizing on the chromosome.
2. Once this unique DNA sequence is known, a fluorescent DNA probe can be constructed.
3. The fluorescent DNA probe is allowed to hybridize with chromosomes prepared for karyotype analysis and thereby visualizes the unique DNA sequence on specific chromosomes.

C. CHROMOSOME PAINTING

1. The chromosome painting technique is based on the construction of fluorescent DNA probes to a wide variety of different DNA fragments from a single chromosome.
2. The fluorescent DNA probes are allowed to hybridize with chromosomes prepared for karyotype analysis and thereby visualize many different loci spanning one whole chromosome (i.e., chromosome paint). Essentially, one whole particular chromosome will fluoresce.

D. SPECTRAL KARYOTYPING OR 24 COLOR CHROMOSOME PAINTING

1. The spectral karyotyping technique is based on chromosome painting whereby DNA probes for all 24 chromosomes are labeled with five different fluorochromes so that each of the 24 chromosomes will have a different ratio of fluorochromes.
2. The different fluorochrome ratios cannot be detected by the naked eye, but computer software can analyze the different ratios and assign a pseudocolor for each ratio.
3. This allows all 24 chromosomes to be painted with a different color. Essentially, all 24 chromosomes will be painted a different color.

E. COMPARATIVE GENOME HYBRIDIZATION (CGH)

1. The CGH technique is based on the competitive hybridization of two fluorescent DNA probes: one DNA probe from a normal cell labeled with a red fluorochrome and the other DNA probe from a tumor cell labeled with a green fluorochrome.
2. The fluorescent DNA probes are mixed together and allowed to hybridize with chromosomes prepared for karyotype analysis.
3. The ratio of red to green signal is plotted along the length of each chromosome as a distribution line. The red/green ratio should be 1:1.
   a. The tumor DNA is missing some of the chromosomal regions present in normal DNA (more red fluorochrome and the distribution line shifts to the left).
   b. The tumor DNA has more of some chromosomal regions than present in normal DNA (more green fluorochrome and the distribution line shifts to the right).

VIII Chromosome Morphology

A. GENERAL FEATURES

1. The appearance of chromosomal DNA can vary considerably in a normal resting cell (e.g., degree of packaging, euchromatin, and heterochromatin) and a dividing cell (e.g., mitosis and meiosis).
2. The pictures of chromosomes seen in karyotype analysis are chromosomal DNA at a particular point in time, that is, arrested at metaphase (or prometaphase) of mitosis. Early metaphase karyograms showed chromosomes as X shaped

because the chromosomes were at a point in mitosis when the protein **cohesin** no longer bound the sister chromatids together, but the centromeres had not yet separated.

3. Modern metaphase karyograms show chromosome as **I** shaped because the chromosomes are at a point in mitosis when the protein **cohesin** still binds the sister chromatids together and the centromeres are not separated. In addition, many modern karyograms are prometaphase karyograms where the chromosomes are **I** shaped.

B. **CHROMOSOME NOMENCLATURE (Figure 1-6)**

1. A chromosome consists of two characteristic parts called **arms**. The short arm is called the **p (petit) arm** and the long arm is called the **q (queue) arm**.

2. The arms can be subdivided into **regions** (counting outward from the centromere), **subregions (bands)**, **subbands** (noted by the addition of a decimal point), and **sub-subbands**.

3. For example, 6p21.34 is read as the short arm of chromosome 6, region 2, and subregion (band) 1, subband 3, and sub-subband 4. This is NOT read as the short arm of chromosome 6, twenty-one point thirty-four.

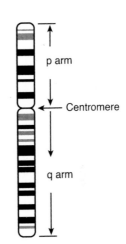

4. In addition, locations on an arm can be referred to in anatomical terms: **proximal** is closer to the centromere and **distal** is farther from the centromere.

● **Figure 1-6 G-banding Pattern of a Metaphase Chromosome.**

5. Figure 1-6 shows the G-banding pattern of a metaphase chromosome along with the centromere, p arm, and q arm.

IX DNA Melting Curve (Figure 1-7)

A. The denaturation of double-stranded DNA to single-stranded DNA can be achieved by **heating** a solution of DNA to a temperature high enough to break the **hydrogen bonds** holding the two complementary strands together.

B. The denaturation of DNA can be followed by measuring the optical density of the DNA at a wavelength of 260 nm (ultraviolet light) which is called the **optical density at 260 nm** (OD_{260}).

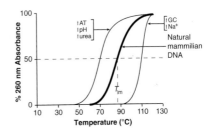

● **Figure 1-7 DNA melting curves.**

C. A measure of double-stranded DNA stability is the **melting temperature** (T_M) which is the temperature where 50% of the double-stranded DNA has been converted to single-stranded DNA.

D. Denaturation of DNA is dependent on

1. **Base composition**

   a. DNA with a high guanine and cytosine content will have a high T_M because guanine and cytosine are connected by three hydrogen bonds ($\uparrow$ **GC content** = $\uparrow T_M$).

   b. DNA with a high adenine and thymine content will have a low T_M because adenine and thymine are connected by two hydrogen bonds ($\uparrow$ **AT content** = $\downarrow T_M$).

2. **Chemical environment**
   a. DNA in the presence of monovalent cations (e.g., Na^+ ions) will have a high T_M because monovalent cations stabilize double-stranded DNA ($\uparrow Na^+ = \uparrow T_M$).
   b. DNA in the presence of alkaline pH will have a low T_M because alkaline pH disrupts the hydrogen bonds ($\uparrow$ **pH** $= \downarrow T_M$).
   c. DNA in the presence of urea will have a low T_M because urea disrupts the hydrogen bonds ($\uparrow$ **urea** $= \downarrow T_M$).

Chapter 2

Chromosome Replication

❶ General Features

A. Chromosome replication occurs during **S phase** of the cell cycle and involves both DNA synthesis and histone synthesis to form chromatin.

B. An **inactive gene** packaged as **heterochromatin** is replicated **late** in S phase. An **active gene** packaged as **euchromatin** is replicated **early** in S phase.

C. DNA-directed DNA polymerases have the following properties:
1. DNA polymerases require a **3′-OH end of a primer strand** as a substrate for strand extension. Therefore, an **RNA primer** (synthesized by a **DNA primase**) is required to provide the free 3′-OH group needed to start DNA synthesis.
2. DNA polymerases copy a DNA template in the **3′ → 5′ direction**, which produces new DNA strand in the **5′ → 3′ direction**.
3. DNA polymerases have **proofreading ability** which depends on 3′ → 5′ **proofreading exonuclease** activity that is associated with the DNA polymerase complex. These are called **high-fidelity DNA polymerases**.

D. DEOXYRIBONUCLEOSIDE 5′-TRIPHOSPHATES (dATP, dTTP, dGTP, dCTP) pair with the corresponding base (A-T, G-C) on the template strand and form a **3′,5′-phosphodiester bond** with the 3′-OH group on the **deoxyribose sugar** which releases a **pyrophosphate**.

E. Chromosome replication is **semiconservative**, which means that double-helix DNA contains one intact parental DNA strand and one newly synthesized DNA strand.

F. Chromosome replication is **bidirectional**, which means that replication begins at a replication origin and simultaneously moves out in both directions from the replication origin.

❷ The Chromosome Replication Process (Figure 2-1)

A. Chromosome replication begins at specific nucleotide sequences located throughout the chromosome called **replication origins**. Eukaryotic DNA contains **multiple replication origins** to ensure rapid DNA synthesis.

B. The enzyme **DNA helicase** recognizes the replication origin and opens up the double helix at that site forming a **replication bubble** with a **replication fork** at each end. The stability of the replication fork is maintained by **single-stranded binding proteins**. The **replisome** refers to a complex molecular machine that carries out DNA replication.

C. As the replication fork moves along the double-stranded DNA, the DNA ahead of the replication fork becomes **overwound** or **positively supercoiled**, whereas the DNA behind the replication fork becomes **underwound** or **negatively supercoiled**. **DNA topoisomerases** solve this problem by altering DNA supercoiling.

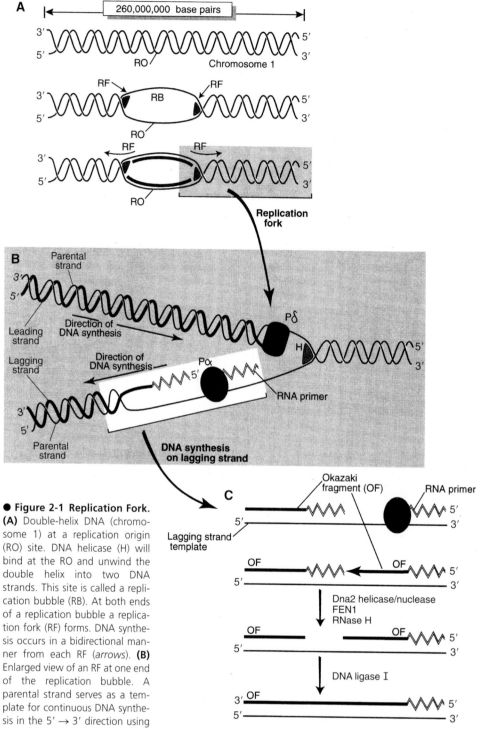

● **Figure 2-1 Replication Fork.**
(A) Double-helix DNA (chromosome 1) at a replication origin (RO) site. DNA helicase (H) will bind at the RO and unwind the double helix into two DNA strands. This site is called a replication bubble (RB). At both ends of a replication bubble a replication fork (RF) forms. DNA synthesis occurs in a bidirectional manner from each RF (*arrows*). **(B)** Enlarged view of an RF at one end of the replication bubble. A parental strand serves as a template for continuous DNA synthesis in the 5′ → 3′ direction using DNA polymerase δ (Pδ). The other parental strand serves as a template for discontinuous DNA synthesis in the 5′ → 3′ direction using DNA polymerase α (Pα). Note that DNA synthesis of the leading and lagging strands is in the 5′ → 3′ direction but physically running in opposite directions. **(C)** DNA synthesis of the lagging strand proceeds differently from that of the leading strand. DNA primase synthesizes RNA primers. DNA polymerase α uses these RNA primers to synthesize DNA fragments called Okazaki fragments (OF). Okazaki fragments end when they run into a downstream RNA primer. Subsequently, DNA repair enzymes remove the RNA primers and replace them with DNA. Finally, DNA ligase joins all the Okazaki fragments together. FEN1 = flap endonuclease 1.

D. A replication fork contains a:

1. Leading strand that is synthesized from the parental strand continuously by **DNA polymerase δ (delta).**

2. Lagging strand that is synthesized from the parental strand discontinuously by **DNA polymerase α (alpha).**

    a. **DNA primase** synthesizes **RNA primers** along the lagging strand.

    b. **DNA polymerase α** uses the RNA primers to synthesize DNA fragments called **Okazaki fragments.** Okazaki fragments end when they run into a downstream RNA primer.

    c. Okazaki fragments contain an RNA/DNA primer that must be removed before the Okazaki fragments can be joined. The RNA/DNA primer is raised into a flap.

    d. **Dna2 helicase/nuclease** and **flap endonuclease 1 (FEN 1)** remove the flap.

    e. **RNase H** degrades the RNA.

    f. **DNA ligase I** subsequently joins all the DNA fragments together.

E. PROKARYOTIC DNA REPLICATION. Prokaryotic (bacterial) DNA replication has some important distinctions compared with eukaryotic DNA replication as follows:

1. DNA polymerase III replicates DNA on both the leading strand and the lagging strand.

2. DNA polymerase I removes RNA primers and replaces them with DNA to form a continuous DNA strand with the Okazaki fragments on the lagging strand.

3. Dna A protein recognizes the replication origin and opens up the double helix at that site forming a **replication bubble.**

4. Okazaki fragments are processed by **DNA polymerase I, RNase,** and **DNA ligase H.**

III   DNA Topoisomerases (Figure 2-2). DNA topoisomerases are enzymes that alter the supercoiling of double-stranded DNA. **Supercoiling** of DNA is a mathematical property representing the sum of the **DNA twists** (the number of helical turns in the DNA) plus the **DNA writhe** (number of times the DNA loops over itself). **Positive supercoiling** refers to overwound DNA. **Negative supercoiling** refers to **underwound** DNA.

A. TYPE I TOPOISOMERASE

1. Type I topoisomerase produces a **transient single-strand nick** in the phosphodiester backbone which allows the DNA on either side of the nick to rotate freely using the phosphodiester bond in the unnicked strand as a **swivel point** and then the nick is resealed. **ATP hydrolysis (energy)** is not required for this process.

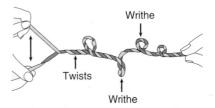
● Figure 2-2 Supercoiling of DNA.

2. Type I topoisomerase **introduces negative supercoiling (or relaxes positive supercoiling).** That is to say, Type I topoisomerase **unwinds DNA.**

3. The chemotherapy drugs **irinotecan** and **topotecan** inhibit Type I topoisomerase in cancer cells.

B. TYPE II TOPOISOMERASE

1. Type II topoisomerase produces a **transient double-strand nick** in the phosphodiester backbone at a site where the DNA loops over itself. Type II topoisomerase breaks one double helix of the loop so that a **DNA gate** is formed, the DNA gate allows the other nearby double helix of the loop to pass through, and then the nick is resealed. **ATP hydrolysis** is required for this process.

2. Type II topoisomerase **introduces negative supercoiling (or relaxes positive supercoiling)**. That is to say, Type II topoisomerase **unwinds DNA.**

3. The chemotherapy drugs **etoposide, teniposide,** and **HU-331** (a quinolone synthesized from cannabidiol) inhibit Type II topoisomerase in cancer cells.

C. DNA GYRASE

1. DNA gyrase is a variant of Type II topoisomerase.

2. DNA gyrase **introduces negative supercoiling (or relaxes positive supercoiling).** That is to say, DNA gyrase unwinds **DNA.**

3. DNA gyrase is found in bacteria and is inhibited by two classes of antibiotics: the **aminocoumarins** (e.g., **novobiocin**) and the **quinolones** (e.g., **ciprofloxacin and nalidixic acid**).

D. REVERSE GYRASE

1. Reverse gyrase is a variant of Type I topoisomerase found in hyperthermophilic bacteria.

2. Reverse gyrase **introduces positive supercoiling.** That is to say, reverse gyrase **winds DNA.**

IV The Telomere

A. The human telomere is a 3–20 kb repeating nucleotide sequence (**TTAGGG**) located at the end of a chromosome.

B. The telomere allows replication of linear DNA to its full length. Since DNA polymerases CANNOT synthesize in the $3' \rightarrow 5'$ direction or start synthesis de novo, removal of the RNA primers will always leave the 5′ end of the lagging strand shorter than the parental strand. If the 5′ end of the lagging strand is not lengthened, a chromosome would get progressively shorter as the cell goes through a number of cell divisions.

C. This problem is solved by a special **RNA-directed DNA polymerase or reverse transcriptase** called **telomerase** (which has an RNA and protein component).

D. The RNA component of telomerase carries an **AAUCCC** sequence (antisense sequence of the TTAGGG telomere) that recognizes the TTAGGG sequence on the parental strand and adds many repeats of TTAGGG to the parental strand.

E. After the repeats of TTAGGG are added to the parental strand, **DNA polymerase α** uses the TTAGGG repeats as a template to synthesize the complementary repeats on the lagging strand. Thus, the lagging strand is lengthened.

F. **DNA LIGASE** joins the repeats to the lagging strand and a **nuclease** cleaves the ends to form double-helix DNA with flush ends.

G. Telomerase is present in human germline cells (i.e., spermatogonia, oogonia) and stem cells (e.g., in skin, bone marrow, and gut), but is absent from most other somatic cells.

V DNA Damage

A. GENERAL FEATURES

1. Chromosomal breakage refers to breaks in chromosomes due to sunlight (or ultraviolet) irradiation, ionizing irradiation, DNA cross-linking agents, or DNA-damaging agents.

2. These insults may cause **depurination of DNA, deamination of cytosine to uracil,** or **pyrimidine dimerization,** which must be repaired by DNA repair enzymes.
3. The normal response to DNA damage is to stall the cell in the G_1 phase of the cell cycle until the damage is repaired.
4. The system that detects and signals DNA damage is a multiprotein complex called **BASC (BRCA1-associated genome surveillance complex).** Some the components of BASC include **ATM (ataxia telangiectasia mutated) protein, BRCA1 protein,** and **BRCA2 protein.**

B. TYPES OF DNA DAMAGE

1. **Depurination.** About 5000 purines (As or Gs) per day are lost from DNA of each human cell when the N-glycosyl bond between the purine and the deoxyribose sugar-phosphate is broken. This is the most frequent type of lesion and leaves the deoxyribose sugar-phosphate with a missing purine base, that is, an apurinic (AP) site.
2. **Deamination of cytosine to uracil.** About 100 cytosines (C) per day are spontaneously deaminated to uracil (U). If the U is not corrected back to a C, then upon replication instead of the occurrence of a correct C-G base pairing, a U-A base pairing will occur.
3. **Pyrimidine dimerization.** Sunlight (UV radiation) can cause covalent linkage of adjacent pyrimidines forming, for example, **thymine dimers.**

VI DNA Repair

A. GENERAL FEATURES

1. DNA repair involves **DNA excision** of the damaged site, **DNA synthesis** of the correct sequence, and **DNA ligation.**
2. DNA repair involves the following enzymes:
   a. **DNA glycosylase** removes damaged bases while leaving the phosphodiester backbone intact which creates an a<u>p</u>urinic/a<u>p</u>yrimidinic (AP) site.
   b. **AP endonuclease** creates a nick in the phosphodiester backbone at the AP site.
   c. **DNA polymerase**
   d. **DNA ligase**

B. TYPES OF DNA REPAIR

1. **Base excision repair.** This type of repair removes a **single damaged base** from a DNA strand.
2. **Nucleotide excision repair.** This type of repair removes a **group of damaged bases** from a DNA strand.
3. **Mismatch repair.** This type of repair removes a **segment of the newly synthesized DNA strand** that contains mismatch base pairs. The newly synthesized DNA strand is recognized by its **lack of methylation.** DNA mismatch repair enzymes are needed for the following reason: If DNA polymerase does not recognize a base pair mismatch during DNA replication and does not correct the base pair mismatch using its $3' \rightarrow 5'$ proofing reading exonuclease activity during replication, then a base pair mismatch occurs that cannot be corrected by DNA polymerase. Therefore, DNA mismatch repair enzymes are necessary to correct base pair mismatches missed by DNA polymerase.

Ⓥⓘⓘ Clinical Considerations

A. XERODERMA PIGMENTOSUM (XP; Figure 2-3)

1. XP is an autosomal recessive genetic disorder caused by mutations in nucleotide **excision repair enzymes**, which results in the inability to remove pyrimidine dimers in individuals who are hypersensitive to **sunlight** (UV radiation).

2. The *XPA* gene and the *XPC* gene are two of the genes involved in the cause of XP. *XPA* gene located on chromosome 9q22.3 encodes for a **DNA repair enzyme**. The **XPC gene** located on chromosome 3p25 also encodes for a **DNA repair enzyme**.

3. **Clinical features include:** sunlight (UV radiation) hypersensitivity with sunburn-like reaction, severe skin lesions around the eyes and eyelids, and malignant skin cancers (basal and squamous cell carcinomas and melanomas) whereby most individuals die by 30 years of age. Figure 2-2 (top) shows a young girl in the early stages of XP with a sunburn-like reaction on the cheeks. Figure 2-2 (bottom) shows a boy in the late stages of XP with malignant skin cancers in the facial area.

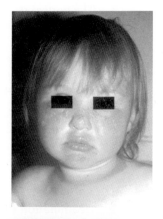
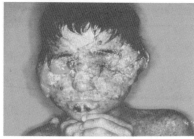

● Figure 2-3 Xeroderma Pigmentosum.

B. COCKAYNE SYNDROME (CS)

1. CS is an autosomal recessive genetic disorder caused by mutations in excision repair enzymes involved in **transcription-coupled** nucleotide excision repair.

2. The *ERCC8* gene and the *ERCC6* gene are two of the genes involved in the cause of CS. The *ERCC8* gene located on chromosome 5 encodes for a <u>e</u>xcision <u>r</u>epair <u>c</u>ross-<u>c</u>omplementing group 8 enzyme. The *ERCC6* gene located on chromosome 10q11 encodes for <u>e</u>xcision <u>r</u>epair <u>c</u>ross-<u>c</u>omplementing group 6 enzyme.

3. **Clinical features include:** sunlight (UV radiation) hypersensitivity, short stature, premature aging, impaired development of nervous system, premature aging, hearing loss, and eye abnormalities (pigmentary retinopathy).

C. ATAXIA-TELANGIECTASIA (AT; Figure 2-4)

1. AT is an autosomal recessive genetic disorder caused by mutations in **DNA recombination repair enzymes** on chromosome 11q22-q23 which results in individuals who are hypersensitive to **ionizing radiation**.

2. The *ATM* gene (AT mutated) is one of the genes involved in the cause of AT. The *ATM* gene located on chromosome 11q22 encodes for a protein where one region resembles a **PI-3 kinase** (phosphatidylinositol-3 kinase) and another region resembles a **DNA repair enzyme/cell cycle checkpoint protein.**

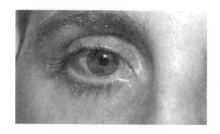
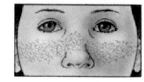

● Figure 2-4 Ataxia-Teleangiectasia.

3. **Clinical features include:** ionizing radiation hypersensitivity; cerebellar ataxia with depletion of Purkinje cells; progressive nystagmus; slurred speech; oculocutaneous telangiectasia (permanent dilation of preexisting small blood vessels creating focal red lesions) initially in the bulbar conjunctiva followed by ear, eyelid, cheeks, and neck; immunodeficiency; and death in the second decade of life. A high frequency of structural rearrangements of chromosomes 7 and 14 is the cytogenetic observation with this disease. Figure 2-4 (top) shows the appearance of telangiectasia of the bulbar conjunctiva. Figure 2-4 (bottom) shows widespread telangiectasia of the cheeks and nose.

D. **HEREDITARY NONPOLYPOSIS COLORECTAL CANCER (HNPCC; or Warthin-Lynch Syndrome)**
    1. HNPCC is an autosomal dominant genetic disorder caused by mutations in **DNA mismatch repair enzymes** which results in the inability to remove single nucleotide mismatches or loops that occur in microsatellite repeat areas.
    2. The four genes involved in the cause of HNPCC include:
        a. **MLH1 gene** located on chromosome 3p21.3, which encodes for DNA mismatch repair protein Mlh1.
        b. **MSH2 gene** located on chromosome 2p22-p21, which encodes for DNA mismatch repair protein Msh2.
        c. **MSH6 gene** located on chromosome 2p16, which encodes for DNA mismatch repair protein Msh6.
        d. **PMS2 gene** located on chromosome 7p22, which encodes for PMS1 protein homolog 2.
    3. These genes are the human homologues to the *Escherichia coli* **mutS** gene and **mutL** gene that code for DNA mismatch repair enzymes.
    4. **Clinical features include:** onset of colorectal cancer at a young age, high frequency of carcinomas proximal to the splenic flexure, multiple synchronous or metachronous colorectal cancers, and presence of extracolonic cancers (e.g., endometrial and ovarian cancer; adenocarcinomas of the stomach, small intestine, and hepatobiliary tract), and account for 3%–5% of all colorectal cancers.

Summary of Chromosome Replication Machinery (Table 2-1)

TABLE 2-1	DNA REPLICATION MACHINERY
Component	**Function**
DNA helicase	Recognizes the replication fork and opens up the double helix
DNA Topoisomerases (in general)	Alter the supercoiling of DNA (in general)
Type I topoisomerase	Introduces negative supercoiling (or relaxes positive supercoiling)
Type II topoisomerase	Introduces negative supercoiling (or relaxes positive supercoiling)
DNA gyrase	Introduces negative supercoiling (or relaxes positive supercoiling)
Revere gyrase	Introduces positive supercoiling
High-Fidelity DNA-Directed DNA Polymerases	
DNA polymerase α	Synthesizes the lagging strand
DNA polymerase β	Repairs DNA by base excision
DNA polymerase γ	Synthesizes mitochondrial DNA
DNA polymerase δ	Synthesizes the leading strand
DNA polymerase ε	Repairs DNA by nucleotide and base excision
Low-Fidelity DNA-Directed DNA Polymerases	
DNA polymerase ζ	
DNA polymerase η	Involved in hypermutation in B and T lymphocytes
DNA polymerase ι	
DNA polymerase μ	
Telomerase*	Lengthens the end of the lagging strand to its full length
DNA primase	Synthesizes short RNA primers
DNA ligase	Catalyzes the formation of the 3′,5′-phosphodiester bond; joins DNA fragments
Single-stranded binding proteins	Maintain the stability of the replication fork

High fidelity = DNA sequence faithfully copied; Low Fidelity = DNA sequence not faithfully copied (error prone).
*Telomerase is an RNA-directed DNA polymerase (or a reverse transcriptase).

Chapter 3

Meiosis and Genetic Recombination

① **Meiosis (Figure 3-1).** Meiosis is a specialized process of cell division (contrasted with mitosis which occurs in somatic cells; see Chapter 10: Cell Cycle) that occurs only in the production of the gametes (i.e., occurs only in the testes and ovary). In general, meiosis consists of two cell divisions (Meiosis I and Meiosis II), but only one round of DNA replication that results in the formation of four gametes, each containing half the number of chromosomes (23 chromosomes) and half the amount of DNA (1 N) found in normal somatic cells (46 chromosomes, 2 N). The various aspects of meiosis compared with mitosis are given in Table 3-1.

A. MEIOSIS I. Events that occur during Meiosis I include

1. **Meiosis S phase (DNA replication)**

2. **Synapsis**
   a. Synapsis refers to the pairing of 46 homologous duplicated chromosomes side by side which occurs only in Meiosis I (not Meiosis II or mitosis).
   b. In female meiosis, each chromosome has a homologous partner whereby the two X chromosomes synapse and crossover just like the other pairs of homologous chromosomes.
   c. In male meiosis, there is a problem because the X and Y chromosomes are very different. However, the X and Y chromosomes do pair and crossover. The pairing of the X and Y chromosomes is an **end-to-end fashion** (rather than along the whole length as for all the other chromosomes) which is made possible by a 2.6-Mb region of sequence homology between the X and Y chromosomes at the tips of their p arms.

3. **Crossover**
   a. Crossover refers to the **equal exchange** of large segments of DNA between the maternal chromatid and paternal chromatid (i.e., nonsister chromatids) at the **chiasma** which occurs during prophase (pachytene) of Meiosis I.
   b. Crossover introduces one **level of genetic variability** among the gametes and occurs by a process called **general recombination.**
   c. During crossover, two other events (i.e., **unequal crossover** and **unequal sister chromatid exchange**) introduce **variable number tandem repeat (VNTR) polymorphisms** into the human nuclear genome.

4. **Alignment.** Alignment refers to the condition whereby the 46 homologous duplicated chromosomes align at the metaphase plate.

5. **Disjunction**
   a. Disjunction refers to the separation of the 46 maternal and paternal homologous duplicated chromosomes from each other into separate secondary gametocytes (*Note*: the **centromeres do not split**).
   b. However, the choice of which maternal or paternal homologous duplicated chromosomes enters the secondary gametocyte is a **random distribution.**

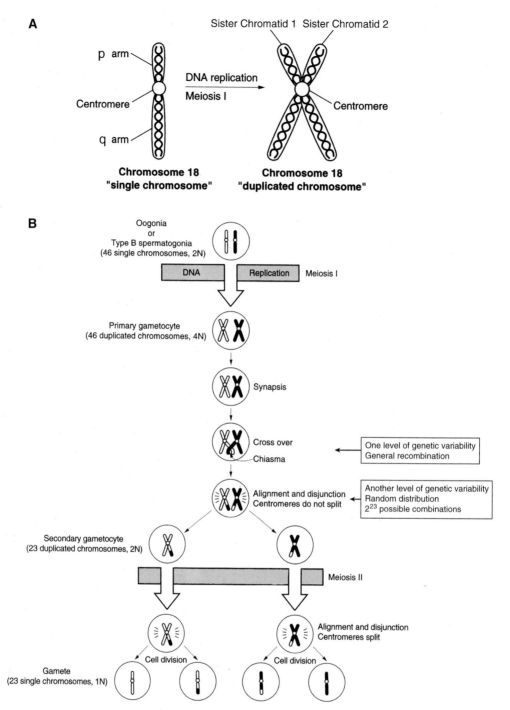

● **Figure 3-1 (A)** Diagram of chromosome 18. The diagram shows chromosome 18 in its "single chromosome" state and "duplicated chromosome" state (that is formed by DNA replication during Meiosis I). It is important to understand that both the "single chromosome" state and "duplicated chromosome" state will be counted as one chromosome 18. As long as the additional DNA in the "duplicated chromosome" is bound at the centromere, the structure will be counted as one chromosome 18 even though it has twice the amount of DNA. The "duplicated chromosome" is often referred to as consisting of two sister chromatids (chromated 1 and chromatid 2). **(B)** Diagram of Meiosis I and Meiosis II. This diagram emphasizes the changes in chromosome number and amount of DNA that occur during gametogenesis. Only one pair of homologous chromosomes is shown (white = maternal origin and black = paternal origin). The point at which DNA crosses over is called the **chiasma.** Segments of DNA are exchanged thereby introducing genetic variability to the gametes. In addition, various cell types along with their appropriate designation of number of chromosomes and amount of DNA is shown.

    c.   There are 2^{23} possible ways the maternal and paternal homologous duplicated chromosomes can be combined. This random distribution of maternal and paternal homologous duplicated chromosomes introduces **another level of genetic variability** among the gametes.

  6. **Cell division:** two secondary gametocytes (23 duplicated chromosomes, 2 N) are formed.

B. **MEIOSIS II.** Events that occur during Meiosis II include

  1. **Synapsis:** absent.

  2. **Crossover:** absent.

  3. **Alignment:** 23 duplicated chromosomes align at the metaphase plate.

  4. **Disjunction:** 23 duplicated chromosomes separate to form 23 single chromosomes when the **centromeres split.**

  5. **Cell division:** gametes (23 single chromosomes, 1 N) are formed.

Ⅱ **Genetic Recombination (Figure 3-2).** For genetic variability to occur, DNA has the ability to undergo rearrangements by a process called **genetic recombination**. There are two types of genetic recombination as indicated below:

A. **GENERAL RECOMBINATION (Figure 3-2A)**

  1. General recombination involves **single-stranded DNA** and requires **DNA sequence homology.** An important example of general recombination occurs during **crossover** when 2 homologous chromosomes pair during the formation of the gametes.

  2. **Rec BCD** protein will make single-strand nicks in DNA to form single-stranded "whiskers."

  3. **SSB** (single-strand binding) proteins stabilize the single-stranded DNA.

  4. **Rec A** protein allows the single strand to invade and interact with the DNA double helix of the other chromosome. This interaction requires DNA sequence homology.

  5. A DNA strand on the homologous chromosome repeats the same process to form an important intermediate structure called a **crossover exchange** (or **Holliday junction**) which consists of two crossing strands and two noncrossing strands.

  6. In a complex process called **resolution** that involves rotation, the DNA strands are cut and DNA repair occurs to produce two homologous chromosomes with exchanged segments of DNA.

B. **SITE-SPECIFIC RECOMBINATION (Figure 3-2B)**

  1. Site-specific recombination involves insertion of **double-stranded DNA.** An important example of site-specific recombination is the insertion of **viral DNA** into host DNA.

  2. Many DNA viruses and other transposable elements encode for a recombination enzyme called **integrase** or **transposase.**

  3. **Integrase** recognizes specific nucleotide sequences (hence the name, site specific) and cuts the viral DNA.

  4. The cut ends of the viral DNA attack and break the host double helix DNA.

  5. The viral DNA is inserted into the host DNA.

  6. Gaps are filled in by DNA repair.

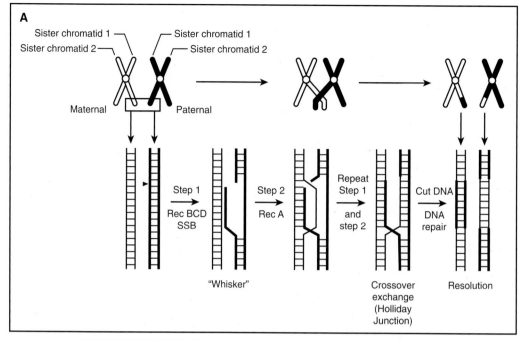

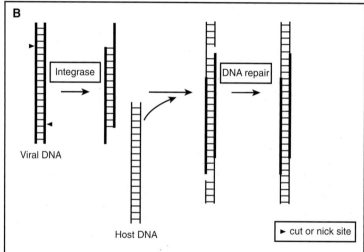

● **Figure 3-2 Types of genetic recombination. (A)** This diagrams shows general recombination that occurs during meiosis. **(B)** This diagram shows site-specific recombination that occurs during DNA viral infection. (▲) Cut or nick sites.

TABLE 3-1	COMPARISON OF MEIOSIS AND MITOSIS
Meiosis	**Mitosis**
Occurs only in the testis and ovary	Occurs in a wide variety of tissues and organs
Produces haploid (23, 1N) gametes (sperm and secondary oocyte)	Produces diploid (46, 2N) somatic daughter cells
Involves two cell divisions and one round of DNA replication	Involves one cell division and one round of DNA replication

Stages of Meiosis
Meiosis I
  Meiosis S Phase (DNA Replication)
  Prophase
    Leptotene (homologue pairing begins; long, thin DNA stands)
    Zygotene (synapsis occurs; synaptonemal complex is formed)
    Pachytene (crossover occurs; short, thick DNA strands)
    Diplotene (chromosomes separate except at centromere)
  Prometaphase
  Metaphase
  Anaphase
  Telophase
 	
Meiosis II (essentially identical to mitosis)
  Prophase
  Prometaphase
  Metaphase
  Anaphase
  Telophase
	Stages of Mitosis
	  Interphase
	    G_0 Phase
	    G_1 Phase
	    S Phase
	    G_2 Phase
	  Prophase
	  Prometaphase
	  Metaphase
	  Anaphase
	  Telophase

Male: Prophase of Meiosis I lasts ~22 days and completes Meiosis II in a few hours Female: Prophase of Meiosis I lasts ~14 years (until puberty) and completes Meiosis II when fertilization occurs	Interphase lasts ~15 hours M phase lasts ~1 hour
Pairing of homologous chromosomes occurs	No pairing of homologous chromosomes
Genetic recombination occurs (exchange of large segments of maternal and paternal DNA via crossover during Meiosis I)	Genetic recombination does not occur
Maternal and paternal homologous chromosomes are randomly distributed among the gametes to ensure genetic variability	Maternal and paternal homologous chromosomes are faithfully distributed among the daughter cells to ensure genetic similarity
Gametes are genetically different	Daughter cells are genetically identical

Chapter 4

The Human Nuclear Genome

❶ General Features (Figure 4-1)

A. The human genome refers to the total DNA content in the cell which is divided into two genomes: the very complex **nuclear genome** and the relatively simple **mitochondrial genome.**

B. The human nuclear genome consists of 24 different chromosomes (22 autosomes; X and Y sex chromosomes).

C. The human nuclear genome codes for ≈30,000 genes (precise number is uncertain) which make up ≈2% of human nuclear genome. Figure 4-1 shows the organization of the human nuclear genome.

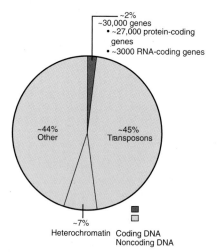

● Figure 4-1 Pie chart indicating the organization of the human nuclear genome.

D. There are ≈27,000 protein-coding genes (i.e., they follow the central dogma of molecular biology: DNA transcribes RNA → mRNA translates protein).

E. There are ≈3000 RNA-coding genes (i.e., they do not follow the central dogma of molecular biology: DNA transcribes RNA → RNA is <u>NOT</u> translated into protein).

F. The fact that the ≈30,000 genes make up only ≈2% of the human nuclear genome means that ≈2% of the human nuclear genome consists of coding DNA and ≈98% of the human nuclear genome consists of noncoding DNA.

G. There is no correspondence between biological complexity of a species and the number of protein-coding genes and RNA-coding genes (i.e., **biological complexity ≠ amount of coding DNA**).

H. There is correspondence between biological complexity of a species and the amount of noncoding DNA (i.e., **biological complexity = amount of noncoding DNA**).

I. To fully understand how heritable traits (both normal and disease related) are passed down, it is important to understand three aspects of the human nuclear genome which include the following:

    1. Protein-coding genes. For decades, protein-coding genes were enshrined as the sole repository of heritable traits. A mutation in a protein-coding gene caused the formation of an abnormal protein and hence an altered trait or disease. Today, we know that protein-coding genes are not the sole repository of heritable traits and that the situation is extremely more complicated involving RNA-coding genes and epigenetic control.

2. **RNA-coding genes.** RNA-coding genes produce **active RNAs** that can profoundly alter normal gene expression and hence produce an altered trait or disease.

3. **Epigenetic control.** Epigenetic control involves chemical **modification of DNA** (e.g., methylation) and **chemical modification of histones** (e.g., acetylation, phosphorylation, and addition of ubiquitin) both of which can profoundly alter normal gene expression and hence produce an altered trait or disease.

Ⅱ Protein-Coding Genes

A. **SIZE.** The size of protein-coding genes varies considerably from the 1.7-kb insulin gene → 45 kb low density lipoprotein (LDL) receptor gene → 2400 kb dystrophin gene.

B. **EXON–INTRON ORGANIZATION**
   1. **Exons (expression sequences)** are coding regions of a gene with an average size of <200 bp.
   2. **Introns (intervening sequences)** are noncoding regions of a gene with a huge variation in size.

C. **REPETITIVE DNA SEQUENCES.** Repetitive DNA sequences may be found in both exons and introns.

D. **CLASSIC GENE FAMILY.** A classic gene family is a group of genes that exhibit a **high degree of sequence homology** over most of the gene length.

E. **GENE SUPERFAMILY.** A gene superfamily is a group of genes that exhibit a **low degree of sequence homology** over most of the gene length. However, there is relatedness in the protein function and structure. Examples of gene superfamilies include the immunoglobulin superfamily, globin superfamily, and the G-protein receptor superfamily.

F. **ORGANIZATION OF GENES IN GENE FAMILIES**
   1. **Cluster.** Genes can be organized as a **tandem repeated array with close clustering** (where the genes are controlled by a single expression control locus) and **compound clustering** (where related and unrelated genes are clustered) all on a single chromosome.
   2. **Dispersed.** Genes can be organized in a dispersed fashion at two or more different chromosome locations all on a single chromosome.
   3. **Multiple clusters.** Genes can be organized in multiple clusters at various chromosome locations and on different chromosomes.

G. **UNPROCESSED PSEUDOGENES, TRUNCATED GENES, INTERNAL GENE FRAGMENTS.** In humans, there is strong selection pressure to maintain the sequence of important genes. So, to propagate evolutionary changes, there is a need for **gene duplication.** The surplus duplicated genes can diverge rapidly, acquire mutations, and either degenerate into nonfunctional pseudogenes or mutate to produce a functional protein that is evolutionary advantageous. As a result of this process, families of protein-coding genes are frequently characterized by the presence of the following:
   1. **Unprocessed pseudogenes** which are defective copies of genes that are not transcribed into mRNA
   2. **Truncated genes** which are portions of genes lacking 5′ or 3′ ends
   3. **Internal gene fragments** which are internal portions of genes

H. PROCESSED PSEUDOGENES

1. Processed pseudogenes are transcribed into mRNA, converted to cDNA by reverse transcriptase, and then the cDNA is integrated into a chromosome.

2. Processed pseudogenes are typically not expressed as proteins because they lack a promoter sequence.

I. RETROGENES

1. Retrogenes are processed pseudogenes where the cDNA integrates into a chromosome near a promoter sequence by chance. If this happens, then a processed pseudogene will express protein.

2. If selection pressure ensures the continued expression of a processed pseudogene, then the processed pseudogene is considered a **retrogene**.

III RNA-Coding Genes

A. RIBOSOMAL RNA (rRNA) GENES

1. There are ~200 copies of rRNA genes which encode for rRNAs that are components of ribosomes used in protein synthesis.

2. The 200 copies of rRNA genes are located in the nucleolus which consists of portions of five pairs of chromosomes (i.e., 13, 14, 15, 21, and 22) that contain the 200 copies of rRNA genes.

3. The rRNA genes are arranged in clusters called **nucleolar organizers** and within the nucleolar organizers the genes are arranged in a **tandem series**.

B. TRANSFER RNA (tRNA) GENES

1. There are 497 tRNA genes which encode for tRNAs that are used in protein synthesis.

C. SMALL NUCLEAR RNA (snRNA) GENES

1. There are ~80 snRNA genes which encode for snRNAs that are components of the major GU-AG spliceosome and minor AU-AC spliceosome used in RNA splicing during protein synthesis.

D. SMALL NUCLEOLAR RNA (snoRNA) GENES

1. The snoRNA genes encode for snoRNAs that direct site-specific base modifications (2'-O-ribose methylation and pseudouridylation) in rRNA.

2. There are two large clusters of snoRNA genes found on chromosome 15q which are paternally imprinted, expressed in the brain and may play a role in the Prader-Willi syndrome.

E. REGULATORY RNA GENES

1. The regulatory RNA genes encode for RNAs that are similar to mRNA.

2. The SRA-1 (steroid receptor activator) RNA gene encodes for SRA-1 RNA that functions as a coactivator of several steroid receptors.

3. The XIST gene encodes for XIST RNA that functions in X chromosome inactivation.

F. MICRO RNA (miRNA) OR SMALL INTERFERING RNA (siRNA) GENES

1. There are ~250 miRNA or siRNA genes which encode for miRNAs or siRNAs that block the expression of other genes.

G. ANTISENSE RNA GENES

1. There are ~1600 antisense RNA genes which encode for antisense RNA that binds to mRNA and physically blocks translation.

H. RIBOSWITCH GENES

1. Riboswitch genes encode for riboswitch RNAs which bind to a target molecule, change shape, and then switch on protein synthesis.

Epigenetic Control. There are two main mechanisms of epigenetic control which include

A. CHEMICAL MODIFICATION OF DNA

1. DNA can be chemically modified by **methylation of cytosine nucleotides** performed by **methylating enzymes.**
2. An increased methylation of a DNA segment will make that DNA segment less likely to be transcribed into RNA, and hence any genes in that DNA segment will be silenced (i.e., ↑ **methylation of DNA = silenced genes**).
3. The mechanism that determines which DNA segments are methylated is unknown.
4. DNA methylation plays a crucial role in the epigenetic phenomenon called **genomic imprinting.**
    a. Genomic imprinting is the differential expression of alleles depending on whether the allele is on the paternal chromosome or the maternal chromosome.
    b. When a gene is imprinted, only the allele on the paternal chromosome is expressed, whereas the allele on the maternal chromosome is silenced (or visa versa).
    c. During male and female gametogenesis, male and female chromosomes must acquire some sort of **imprint** that signals the difference between paternal and maternal alleles.
    d. The role of genomic imprinting is highlighted by several rare diseases like Prader-Willi syndrome, Angelman syndrome, Beckwith-Wiedemann syndrome, and hydatidiform moles that show abnormal DNA methylation patterns.

B. CHEMICAL MODIFICATION OF HISTONES

1. Histone proteins can be chemically modified by **acetylation, methylation, phosphorylation,** or **addition of ubiquitin** (all of which are sometimes called **epigenetic marks** or **epigenetic tags**).
2. An increased acetylation of histone proteins will make a DNA segment more likely to be transcribed into RNA and hence any genes in that DNA segment will be expressed (i.e., ↑ **acetylation of histones = expressed genes**).
3. The mechanism that determines the location and combination of epigenetic tags is unknown.

 Noncoding DNA

A. SATELLITE DNA

1. Satellite DNA is composed of very large-sized blocks (100 kb → several Mb) of tandem-repeated noncoding DNA.
2. **Large-scale variable number tandem repeat (VNTR) polymorphisms** are typically found in satellite DNA.
3. The function of satellite DNA is not known.

B. MINISATELLITE DNA

1. Minisatellite DNA is composed of moderately sized blocks (0.1 kb → 20 kb) of tandem-repeated noncoding DNA.
2. **Simple VNTR polymorphisms** are typically found in minisatellite DNA.
3. Types of minisatellite DNA include
    a. Hypervariable **minisatellite DNA** consists of a 9–64-bp repeat unit and is found near the telomere and other chromosomal locations. Hypervariable minisatellite DNA is a "hotspot" for genetic recombination, is used as a genetic marker, and is used in DNA fingerprinting.

b. **Telomeric DNA** consists of a 6-bp repeat unit and is found at the end of all chromosomes. Telomeric DNA allows the replication of linear DNA of the lagging strand during chromosome replication.

C. MICROSATELLITE DNA (SIMPLE SEQUENCE REPEAT OR SHORT TANDEM REPEATS)

1. Microsatellite DNA is composed of small-sized blocks (1–6 bp) of **tandem-repeated noncoding DNA**. The most common microsatellite in humans is a $(CA)_n$ repeat where $n = 10$–100.

2. The length of microsatellite DNA is highly variable from person to person, but the length of microsatellite DNA is constant in each person. Consequently, microsatellite DNA can be used as a molecular marker in determining paternity and population genetic studies.

3. **Microsatellite instability** refers to a condition whereby microsatellite DNA is abnormally lengthened or shortened due to defects in the DNA repair process.

4. Microsatellite instability is a hallmark feature in **hereditary nonpolyposis colorectal cancer (HNPCC or Warthin-Lynch syndrome)**. All HNPCC tumors show microsatellite DNA throughout the entire genome that has abnormally lengthened or shortened. This microsatellite instability is caused by mutations in genes for **DNA mismatch repair enzymes** (Mlh1, Msh2, and Msh6).

D. TRANSPOSONS (TRANSPOSABLE ELEMENTS; "JUMPING GENES").
Transposons are composed of **interspersed repetitive noncoding DNA** that make up an incredible **45% of the human nuclear genome**. Transposons are mobile DNA sequences that jump from one place in the genome to another (called **transposition**).

1. **Types of transposons**
    a. **Short interspersed nuclear elements (SINEs).** SINEs (~100–400 bps) have been very successful in colonizing the human genome. SINEs are generally transcriptionally active only under stressful situations whereby SINE RNAs promote protein synthesis under stress. The **Alu repeat** (280 bp) is a SINE that is the **most abundant sequence in the human genome**. When Alu repeats are located within genes, they are confined to introns and other untranslated regions.
    b. **Long interspersed nuclear elements (LINEs).** LINE 1 (~6.1 kb) is the **most important human transposon** in that it is still actively transposing (jumping) and occasionally causes disease by disrupting important functioning genes. LINE 1 accounts for almost all the reverse transcriptase activity in the human genome and allows for the retrotransposition and the creation of processed pseudogenes and retrogenes.
    c. **Long terminal repeat (LTR) transposons.** LTR transposons are **retrovirus-like elements** which are flanked by **long terminal repeats (LTRs)** that contain transcriptional regulatory elements. The **endogenous retroviral sequences (ERV)** are LTR transposons that contain the **gag gene** and **pol gene** which encode for a **protease, reverse transcriptase, RNAase H, and integrase**.
    d. **DNA transposons.** DNA transposons contain terminal inverted repeats and encode for the enzyme **transposase** which is used in transposition. Most DNA transposons in humans are no longer active (i.e., they do not jump) and therefore are considered **transposon fossils**.

2. **Mechanism of transposition.** Transposable elements jump either as double-stranded DNA using conservative **transposition** or through an RNA intermediate using **retrotransposition**.

a. **Conservative transposition (Figure 4-2)**. In conservative transposition, the **transposon (T)** located on a **host chromosome** jumps as double-stranded DNA. **Transposase** (encoded in the DNA of the transposon) cuts the transposable element at a site marked by **inverted repeat DNA sequences**. The transposon is inserted into a new location on a **target chromosome**. And the host chromosome undergoes **DNA repair**. This mechanism is similar to the mechanism that a **DNA virus** uses in its life cycle to transform host DNA.

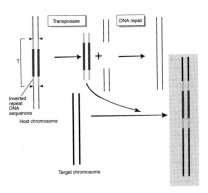

● **Figure 4-2 Conservative Transposition.**

b. **Retrotransposition (Figure 4-3)**. In retrotransposition, the **transposon (T)** undergoes **transcription** which produces an **RNA copy** that encodes a **reverse transcriptase (RT)** enzyme. The reverse transcriptase makes a double-stranded DNA copy of the transposon from the RNA copy. The transposon is inserted into a new location on a **target chromosome** using the enzyme **integrase**. This mechanism is similar to the mechanism that an **RNA virus (retrovirus)** uses in its life cycle to transform host DNA.

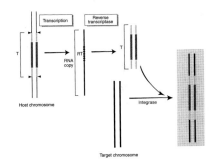

● **Figure 4-3 Retrotransposition.**

3. **Transposons and genetic variability.** The main purpose of transposons is to affect the genetic variability of the organism. Transposons can do this in several ways:

a. **Mutation at the former site of the transposon (Figure 4-4)**. After the transposon **(T)** is cut out of its site in the **host chromosome** by **transposase**, the host chromosome undergoes **DNA repair**. A mutation **(X)** may arise at the repair site.

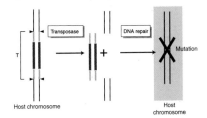

● **Figure 4-4 Mutation at Former Site.**

b. **Level of gene expression (Figure 4-5).** If the **transposon (T)** moves to the **target DNA** near an **active gene**, the transposon may cause a **change in gene expression.** Although most of these changes in gene expression would be detrimental to the organism, some of the changes over time might be beneficial and then spread through the population.

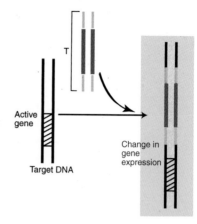

● Figure 4-5 Level of Gene Expression.

c. **Gene inactivation (Figure 4-6).** If the **transposon (T)** moves to the **target DNA** in the middle of an **active gene,** the active gene will be mutated and become an **inactive gene.**

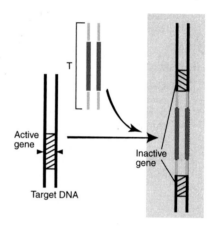

● Figure 4-6 Gene Inactivation.

d. **Gene transfer (Figure 4-7).** If two transposons happen to be close to one another, the transposition mechanism may cut the ends of two different transposons. This mechanism is especially important in **development of antibiotic resistance** in bacteria. If the **bacterial DNA** between to the **two transposons (T)** contains the **gene for tetracycline resistance (Tet^R),** the Tet^R gene may insert into **phage DNA.** The phage DNA with the Tet^R gene infects other bacteria and confers tetracycline resistant.

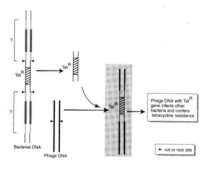

● Figure 4-7 Gene Transfer.

Chapter 5

The Human Mitochondrial Genome

① General Features (Figure 5-1)

A. The human mitochondrial genome consists of mitochondrial DNA (mtDNA) arranged as a **circular piece of double-stranded DNA (H strand and L strand)** consisting of 16,569 base pairs and is located within the **mitochondrial matrix**.

B. In contrast to the human nuclear genome, mtDNA is not protected by histones (i.e., **histone free**).

C. The human mitochondrial genome codes for **37 genes** which make up ≈93% of the human mitochondrial genome.

D. There are **13 protein-coding genes** and **24 RNA-coding genes**.

E. The fact that the 37 genes make up ≈93% of the human mitochondrial genome means that ≈93% of the human mitochondrial genome consists of coding DNA and ≈7% of the human mitochondrial genome consists of noncoding DNA (compare with the human nuclear genome, Chapter 4).

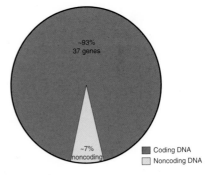

● **Figure 5-1** Pie chart indicating the organization of the human mitochondrial genome.

F. All human mtDNA genes **contain only exons** (i.e., no introns are present).

G. The human mitochondrial genome is **maternally inherited** (i.e., both males and females inherit mtDNA from the mother, but males do not transmit their mtDNA to subsequent generations). During fertilization and zygote formation, the sperm contributes its nuclear genome but not its mitochondrial genome because all sperm mitochondria degenerate. Consequently, the mitochondrial genome of the zygote is determined exclusively by the mitochondria found in the cytoplasm of the unfertilized secondary oocyte.

② The 13 Protein-Coding Genes (Figure 5-2, Table 5-1). The protein-coding genes encode for 13 proteins that are not complete enzymes but are **subunits of multimeric enzyme complexes** used in electron transport and ATP synthesis. These 13 proteins are synthesized on mitochondrial ribosomes.

③ The 24 RNA-Coding Genes (Figure 5-2, Table 5-1). The RNA-coding genes encode for 24 RNAs.

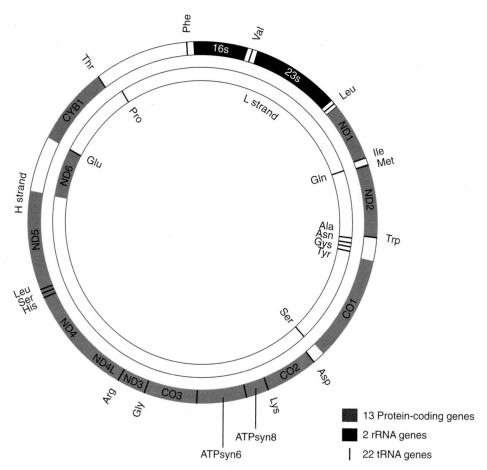

● **Figure 5-2 Location of mtDNA genes and their gene products.** ND1, ND2, ND3, ND4L, ND4, ND5, ND6 = genes for the seven subunits of the NADH dehydrogenase complex; CO1, CO2, CO3 = genes for the three subunits of the cytochrome oxidase complex; ATP synthase 6, ATP synthase 8 = genes for the two subunits of the F_0 ATPase complex; CYB1 = gene for the one subunit (cytochrome b) of ubiquinone-cytochrome c oxidoreductase complex; Phe = phenylalanine tRNA gene; Val = valine tRNA gene; Leu = leucine tRNA gene; Ile = isoleucine tRNA gene; Met = methionine tRNA gene; Trp = tryptophan tRNA gene; Asp = asparagine tRNA gene; Lys = lysine tRNA gene; Gly = glycine tRNA gene; Arg = arginine tRNA gene; His = histidine tRNA gene; Ser = serine tRNA gene; Thr = threonine tRNA gene; Pro = proline tRNA gene; Glu = glutamic acid tRNA gene; Tyr = tyrosine tRNA gene; Cys = cysteine tRNA gene; Asn = asparagine tRNA gene; Ala = alanine tRNA gene; Gln = glutamine tRNA gene; 16S = 16S rRNA gene; 23S = 23S rRNA gene; rRNA = ribosomal RNA; tRNA = transfer RNA.

TABLE 5-1	MITOCHONDRIAL PROTEIN-CODING AND RNA-CODING GENES
13 Protein-coding genes	Seven subunits of the NADH dehydrogenase complex (i.e., ND1, ND2, ND3, ND4L, ND4, ND5, and ND6; Complex I); three subunits of the cytochrome oxidase complex (i.e., CO1, CO2, and CO3; Complex IV); two subunits of the F_0 ATPase complex (i.e., ATP synthase 6 and ATP synthase 8); one subunit (cytochrome b) of ubiquinone-cytochrome c oxidoreductase complex (i.e., CYB1; Complex III)
24 RNA-coding genes	2 rRNAs (16S and 23S) 22 tRNAs (corresponding to each amino acid)

Ⅳ Other Mitochondrial Proteins

A. All other mitochondrial proteins (e.g., enzymes of the citric acid cycle, DNA polymerase, RNA polymerase) are **encoded by nuclear DNA, synthesized on cytoplasmic ribosomes,** and then **imported into the mitochondria.**

B. The importation of proteins into mitochondria is assisted by **chaperone proteins** (**cytoplasmic hsp70, matrix hsp70, and hsp60**), which keep the protein in an **unfolded state** during importation.

C. The unfolded proteins enter the mitochondria through an **import channel** called ISP42.

Ⅴ Mitochondrial Diseases.

In general, mitochondrial diseases show a wide degree of severity among affected individuals. This variability is caused, in part, to the mixture of normal and mutant mtDNA present in a particular cell type (called **heteroplasmy**). When a cell undergoes mitosis, **mitochondria segregate randomly** in the daughter cells. This means that one daughter cell may receive mostly mutated mtDNA and the other daughter cell mostly normal mtDNA. Mitochondrial disorders show a **threshold level** where a critical level of mutated mitochondria must be reached before clinical symptoms appear. A woman who has not reached the threshold level can still have affected children. In addition, mitochondrial diseases affect tissues that have a **high requirement for ATP** (e.g., nerve and skeletal muscle). Mitochondrial diseases include the following:

A. MYOCLONIC EPILEPSY WITH RAGGED RED FIBERS SYNDROME (MERRF)
1. MERRF is a mitochondrial genetic disorder caused by a mutation in the $tRNA^{Lys}$ **gene** whereby a A → G transition occurs at **nucleotide position 8344 (A8344G).**
2. The mutated $tRNA^{Lys}$ causes a **premature termination of translation** of the amino acid chain (the amount and the aminoacylation activity of the mutated $tRNA^{Lys}$ is not affected).
3. Mitochondrial enzymes with large number lysine residues will have a low probability of being completely synthesized. In this regard, **NADH dehydrogenase (Complex I)** and **cytochrome oxidase (Complex IV)** both of which have a large number of lysine residues have been shown to be synthesized at very low rates.
4. Heteroplasmy is common and expression of the disease is highly variable.
5. **Clinical features include** myoclonus (muscle twitching), seizures, cerebellar ataxia, dementia, and mitochondrial myopathy (abnormal mitochondria within skeletal muscle that impart an irregular shape and blotchy red appearance to the muscle cells, hence the term ragged red fibers).

B. LEBER'S HEREDITARY OPTIC NEUROPATHY (LHON)
1. LHON is a mitochondrial genetic disorder caused by three mtDNA missense mutations which account for 90% of all cases worldwide and are therefore designated as **primary LHON mutations.**
2. The primary LHON mutations include the following:
   a. A mutation in the **ND4 gene** (which encodes for subunit 4 of NADH dehydrogenase; Complex I) whereby a A → G transition occurs at **nucleotide position 11778 (A11778G).** This is the most common cause (≈50% of all LHON cases) of LHON.
   b. A mutation in the **ND1 gene** (which encodes for subunit 1 of NADH dehydrogenase; Complex I) whereby a G → A transition occurs at **nucleotide position 3460 (G3460A).**
   c. A mutation in the **ND 6 gene** (which encodes for subunit 6 of NADH dehydrogenase; Complex I) whereby a T → C transition occurs at **nucleotide position 14484 (T14484C).**

3. All three primary LHON mutations **decrease production of ATP** such that the demands of a very active neuronal metabolism cannot be met and suggest a common disease-causing mechanism.

4. Heteroplasmy is rare and expression of the disease is fairly uniform. Consequently, the family pedigree of LHON demonstrates a typical of mitochondrial inheritance pattern.

5. **Clinical features include** progressive optic nerve degeneration that results clinically in blindness, blurred vision, or loss of central vision; telangiectatic microangiopathy; disk pseudoedema; vascular tortuosity; onset occurs at ≈ 20 years of age with precipitous vision loss; and affect males far more often than females for some unknown reason.

C. KEARNS-SAYRE SYNDROME (KS)

1. KS is a mitochondrial genetic disorder caused by **partial deletions of mitochondrial DNA (delta-mtDNA)** and **duplication of mitochondrial DNA (dup-mtDNA)**. The partial deletions of mtDNA have been associated with a marked reduction in the enzymatic activity of NADH dehydrogenase (Complex I), succinate dehydrogenase (Complex II), ubiquinone-cytochrome c oxidoreductase (Complex III), and cytochrome oxidase (Complex IV).

2. Heteroplasmy is common and expression of the disease is highly variable.

3. **Clinical features include** chronic progressive external ophthalmoplegia (degeneration of the motor nerves of the eye), pigmentary degeneration of the retina ("salt and pepper" appearance), heart block, short stature, gonadal failure, diabetes mellitus, thyroid disease, deafness, vestibular dysfunction, and cerebellar ataxia and onset occurs at ≈ 20 years of age.

D. MITOCHONDRIAL MYOPATHY, ENCEPHALOPATHY, LACTIC ACIDOSIS, AND STROKE-LIKE EPISODES SYNDROME (MELAS)

1. MELAS is a mitochondrial genetic disorder caused by a mutation in the $tRNA^{Leu}$ gene whereby a A $\rightarrow$ G transition occurs at **nucleotide position 3243 (A3243G)**.

2. The mutated $tRNA^{Leu}$ causes a reduction in the amount and the aminoacylation of the mutated $tRNA^{Leu}$, a reduction in the association of mRNA with ribosomes, and altered incorporation of leucine into mitochondrial enzymes.

3. Mitochondrial enzymes with a large number of leucine residues will have a low probability of being completely synthesized. In this regard, cytochrome oxidase (Complex IV) has been shown to be synthesized at very low rates.

4. Heteroplasmy is common and expression of the disease is highly variable.

5. **Clinical features include** mitochondrial myopathy, encephalopathy, lactic acidosis, and stroke-like episodes.

Chapter 6

Protein Synthesis

I General Features

A. The flow of genetic information in a cell is almost exclusively in one direction: **DNA → RNA → protein.**

B. The flow of genetic information follows a **colinearity principle** in that a *linear sequence* of nucleotides in DNA is decoded to give a *linear sequence* of nucleotides in RNA which is decoded to give a *linear sequence* of amino acids in a protein.

C. This flow involves three main successive steps called **transcription, processing the RNA transcript,** and **translation.**

II Transcription

A. TRANSCRIPTION IN GENERAL

1. Transcription is the mechanism by which the cell copies **DNA into RNA** and occurs in the **nucleus.**
2. During transcription, the double helix DNA is unwound and the **DNA template strand** forms transient **RNA–DNA hybrid** with the growing RNA transcript. The other DNA strand is called the **DNA nontemplate strand.**
3. DNA sequences which flank the gene sequence at the 5′ end of the template strand are called **upstream sequences.** DNA sequences which flank the gene sequence at the 3′ end of the template strand are called **downstream sequences.**
4. Transcription is carried out by **DNA-directed RNA polymerase** that copies a DNA template strand in the **3′ → 5′ direction** which in turn produces an RNA transcript in the **5′ → 3′ direction.**
5. RNA polymerase differs from DNA polymerase in that RNA polymerase does *not* need a primer and does *not* have 3′ → 5′ proofreading exonuclease activity.
6. There are three RNA polymerases as follows:
   a. **RNA polymerase I** produces 45S rRNA.
   b. **RNA polymerase II** produces an **RNA transcript that is further processed into mRNA** used in protein synthesis.
   c. **RNA polymerase III** produces **5S rRNA, tRNA, some snRNAs, snoRNA, and miRNA (microRNA).**

B. TRANSCRIPTION IN PROTEIN SYNTHESIS (Figure 6-1).

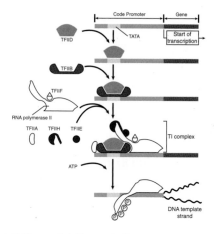

● **Figure 6-1 Transcription.**

1. In protein synthesis, RNA polymerase II produces an RNA transcript by a complex process that involves a number of **general transcription factors** called TFIIs (transcription factors for RNA polymerase II).

2. **TFIID** binds to the TATA box which then allows the adjacent binding of **TFIIB**.

3. The next step involves **TFIIA, TFIIE, TFIIF,** and **TFIIH,** and **RNA polymerase II** engaged to the promoter forming a **transcription initiation (TI) complex.**

4. The TI complex must gain access to the DNA template strand at the transcription start site which is accomplished by TFIIH (a **DNA helicase**).

5. TFIIH also contains a **protein kinase** that phosphorylates (P) RNA polymerase II so that RNA polymerase II is released from the TI complex.

6. The TI complex will produce only a **basal level of transcription** or **constitutive expression.** Other factors called *cis*-acting DNA sequences and *trans*-acting proteins are necessary for increased transcription levels.

III Processing the RNA Transcript into mRNA.

A cell involved in protein synthesis will use RNA polymerase II to transcribe a protein-coding gene into an **RNA transcript** that must be further processed into mRNA. This processing involves

A. **RNA CAPPING** is the addition of a **7-methylguanosine** to the first nucleotide at the 5′ end of the RNA transcript. RNA capping functions to protect the RNA transcript from exonuclease attack, to facilitate transport from the nucleus to the cytoplasm, to facilitate RNA splicing, and to attach the mRNA to the 40S subunit of the ribosome.

B. **RNA POLYADENYLATION** is the addition of a **poly-A tail** (about 200 repeated AMPs) to the **3′ end** of the RNA transcript. The **AAUAAA sequence** is a **polyadenylation signal sequence** which signals the 3′ cleavage of the RNA transcript. After 3′ cleavage, polyadenylation occurs. RNA polyadenylation functions to protect against degradation, to facilitate transport from the nucleus to the cytoplasm, and to enhance recognition of the mRNA by the ribosomes.

C. RNA SPLICING

1. RNA splicing is a process whereby all **introns (noncoding regions; intervening sequences)** are removed from the RNA transcript and all **exons (coding regions; expression sequences)** are joined together within the RNA transcript.

2. RNA splicing requires that the intron/exon boundaries (or **splice junctions**) be recognized. In most cases, introns start with a GT sequence and end with an AG sequence (called the **GT–AG rule**).

3. RNA splicing is carried out by a large RNA–protein complex called the **spliceosome** which consists of **five types of snRNAs (small nuclear RNA)** and >50 different proteins. Each snRNA is complexed to specific proteins to form **small nuclear ribonucleoprotein particles (snRNPs)**.

4. The RNA portion of the snRNPs hybridizes to a nucleotide sequence that marks the intron site (GT–AG rule), whereas the protein portion cuts out the intron and rejoins the RNA transcript. This produces mRNA that can leave the nucleus and be translated in the cytoplasm.

5. There are two type of spliceosome: the **major GU–AG spliceosome** which splices GT–AG introns and the **minor AU–AC spliceosome** which splices the rare class of AT–AC introns.

IV **Translation (Figure 6-2)** is the mechanism by which only the **centrally located nucleotide sequence of mRNA** is translated into the **amino acid sequence of a protein** and occurs in the **cytoplasm**. The end or flanking sequences of the mRNA (called the **5′ and 3′ untranslated regions, 5′UTR and 3′UTR**) are not translated. Translation decodes a set of **three** nucleotides (called a **codon**) into **one** amino acid (e.g., GCA codes for alanine, UAC codes for tyrosine). The code is said to be **redundant** which means that more than one codon specifies a particular amino acid (e.g., GCA, GCC, GCG, and GCU all specify alanine and UAC and UAU both specify tyrosine).

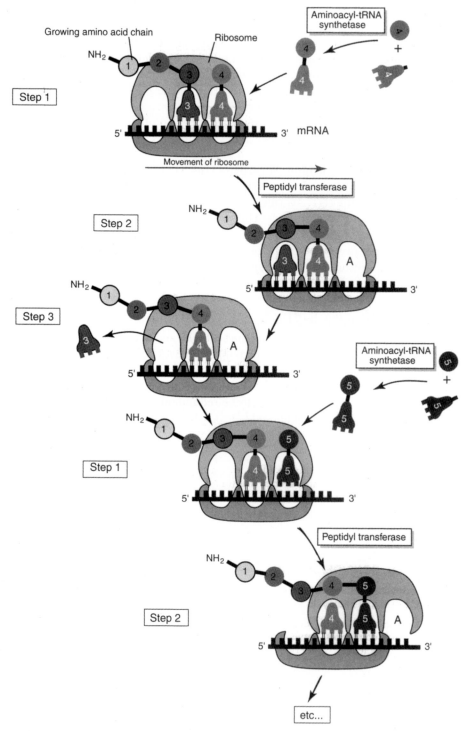

● **Figure 6-2 Translation.** This diagram joins the process of translation at a point where three amino acids have already been linked together (amino acids 1, 2, and 3). The process of translation is basically a three-step process that is repeated over and over during the synthesis of a protein. The enzyme aminoacyl-tRNA synthetase links a specific amino acid with its specific tRNA. In step 1, the tRNA and amino acid complex 4 binds to the A site on the ribosome. Note that the direction of movement of the ribosome along the mRNA is in a 5′ → 3′ direction. In step 2, the enzyme peptidyl transferase forms a peptide bond between amino acid 3 and amino acid 4 and the small subunit of the ribosome reconfigures so that the A site is vacant. In step 3, the used tRNA 3 is ejected and the ribosome is ready for tRNA and amino acid complex 5.

A. Translation uses **transfer RNA (tRNA; Figure 6-3)**. tRNA is a cloverleaf structure consisting of about 75–90 nucleotides and has four arms. The **acceptor arm** contains the **amino acid-binding site**, whereby the amino acid covalently binds at the CCA 3′ end. The **anticodon arm** contains the anticodon trinucleotide in the center of the loop that base pairs with the codon on mRNA. The anticodon arm demonstrates **tRNA wobble**, whereby the normal A-U and G-C pairing is required only in the first two base positions of the codon, but variability or wobble occurs at the third position. The **TψC arm** is defined by this trinucleotide of thymine (T), ψ (pseudouridine; 5-ribosyl uracil), and cytosine (C). tRNA is the only RNA where thymine is present. The **D arm** is named because it contains 5,6-dihydrouridine (D) residues. ψ = pseudouridine (5-ribosyl uracil) m^5 C = 5-methylcytidine m^1 A = 1-methyladenosine D = 5,6-dihydrouridine.

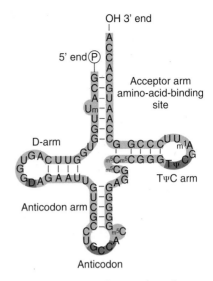

● **Figure 6-3 Transfer RNA (tRNA).**

B. Translation uses the enzyme **aminoacyl-tRNA synthetase** which links an amino acid to tRNA. **tRNA charging** refers to the fact that the amino acid–tRNA bond contains the energy for the formation of the peptide bond between amino acids. There is a specific aminoacyl-tRNA synthetase for each amino acid. Because there are 20 different amino acids, there are 20 different aminoacyl-tRNA synthetase enzymes.

C. Translation uses the enzyme **peptidyl transferase** which participates in forming the peptide bond between amino acids of the growing protein.

D. Translation requires the use of ribosomes which are large RNA–protein complexes that consist of a 40S subunit (consisting of 18S rRNA and ~30 ribosomal proteins) and a 60S subunit (consisting of 5S rRNA, 5.8 rRNA, 28S rRNA, and ~50 ribosomal proteins). The ribosome moves along the mRNA in a **5′ → 3′ direction** such that the **NH2-terminal end** of a protein is synthesized **first** and the **COOH-terminal end** of a protein is synthesized **last**.

E. Translation begins with the start **codon AUG** that codes for **methionine** (the optimal initiation codon recognition sequence is **GCACCAUGG**) so that all newly synthesized proteins have methionine as their first (or NH2 terminal) amino acid which is usually removed later by a protease.

F. Translation terminates at the **stop codon (UAA, UAG, UGA)**. The stop codon binds **release factors** that cause the protein to be released from the ribosome into the cytoplasm.

V Clinical Considerations

A. SYSTEMIC LUPUS ERYTHEMATOSUS (SLE)

1. SLE is a chronic autoimmune disease that affects the blood, joints, skin, and kidneys. SLE occurs predominately in **women of childbearing age**.

2. SLE pathogenesis involves polyclonal B cell activation, sustained estrogen activity, and environmental factors such as the sun or the drug **procainamide (drug-induced SLE)**.

3. Laboratory findings include

  a. **Anti-double-stranded DNA antibodies.**

   b. **Anti-Sm antibodies.** The S̲m̲ith antigen is a protein that keeps DNA in its cor-
       rect shape.
   c. **Anti-SS-A (Ro) antibodies.** The S̲jogren s̲yndrome A̲ antigen is a protein asso-
       ciated with small RNAs called scYRNAs which are present in both the cyto-
       plasm and nucleus.
   d. **Anti-snRNP antibodies.** S̲mall n̲uclear r̲ibo̲nucleoproteins that are used in
       RNA splicing were first characterized by using antibodies from SLE patients.
4. **Clinical findings include** autoimmune hemolytic anemia, thrombocytopenia,
   leukopenia, lymphadenopathy, small joint inflammation, malar butterfly rash, diffuse proliferative glomerulonephritis, pericarditis, Libman-Sacks endocarditis, lung
   interstitial fibrosis, and pregnancy-related complete heart block in newborns
   caused by anti–SS-A (Ro) antibodies crossing the placenta.

B. β-THALASSEMIA

1. β-Thalassemia is an autosomal recessive genetic disorder caused by >200 missense
    or frameshift mutations in the *HBB* gene on **chromosome 11p15.5** for the **β-globin
    subunit of hemoglobin.**
2. β-Thalassemia is defined by the absence or reduced synthesis of β-globin subunits
    of hemoglobin.
    a. A β^0 **mutation** refers to a mutation that causes the absence of β-globin sub-
        units. The **β-globin gene** has three exons and two introns. The introns con-
        tain a **G–T sequence** that are responsible for correct RNA splicing to occur
        and form normal β-globin mRNA. In β^0-thalassemia, the G–T sequence is mu-
        tated to A–T such that correct RNA splicing does NOT occur and the defec-
        tive β-globin mRNA cannot be translated into β-globin protein. β^0-thalassemia
        produces severe anemia in the affected individuals.
    b. A β^+ **mutation** refers to a mutation that causes the reduced synthesis of β-
        globin subunits. It should be noted that the clinical amount of β-globin sub-
        units of hemoglobin is due to **two (2) alleles.**
3. The mutations in the *HBB* gene result in the **reduced amounts of HbA (Hb $\alpha_2\beta_2$)**
    because there is reduced synthesis of β-globin subunits which are found only in HbA.
4. Heterozygote carriers of β-thalassemia are often referred to as having **thalassemia
    minor.**
    a. Thalassemia minor results from the inheritance of a β^+ mutation of one β-
        globin allele (β^+/normal β).
    b. **Clinical features include** individuals who are asymptomatic with very mild or
        absent anemia, but red blood cell abnormalities may be seen.
5. **Prevalence.** The prevalence of β-thalassemia is very high in the African, Mediter-
    ranean, Arabic, Indian, and Southeast Asian populations. The prevalence of β-
    thalassemia is 1/7 births in Cyprus and 1/8 births in Sardinia.
6. There are two clinically significant forms of β-thalassemia:
    a. **Thalassemia major.** Thalassemia major results from the inheritance of a β^0 mu-
        tation of both β-globin alleles (β^0/β^0) and is the most severe form of β-tha-
        lassemia. An **excess of α-globin subunits** form insoluble inclusion bodies within
        mature red blood cell precursors. **Clinical features include** microcytic hypochro-
        matic hemolytic anemia, abnormal peripheral blood smear with nucleated red
        blood cells, reduced amounts of HbA, severe anemia, hepatosplenomegaly, fail
        to thrive, become progressively pale, regular blood transfusion are necessary, and
        usually come to medical attention between 6 months → 2 years of age.
    b. **Thalassemia intermedia.** Thalassemia intermedia results from the inheritance
        of a β^0 mutation of one β-globin allele (β^0/normal β) and is a less severe form
        of β-thalassemia. **Clinical features include** a mild hemolytic anemia, individ-
        uals are at risk for iron overload, regular blood transfusions are rarely neces-
        sary, and usually come to medical attention by >2 years of age.

Chapter 7

Control of Gene Expression

I — General Features

A. HOUSEKEEPING GENES. All cells in the human body contain **housekeeping genes** which are expressed and produce **housekeeping proteins** that are used for many functions common to all cells (e.g., enzymes for metabolic processes, cytoskeleton proteins, and proteins essential to the endoplasmic reticulum and Golgi).

B. However, differentiated cells produce **specialized proteins** (e.g., hepatocytes produce Factor VIII and the pancreatic beta cells produce insulin).

C. Because all cells in the human body contain identical DNA, the key cell biological question is why do hepatocytes produce Factor VIII and not insulin? Or, why do pancreatic beta cells produce insulin and not Factor VIII? The answers to these questions fall into the area of **gene expression** or **gene regulation**.

II — Mechanism of Gene Expression (Figure 7-1).

The mechanism of gene expression employs the use of both *cis*-acting **DNA sequences** and *trans*-acting **proteins**.

A. *CIS*-ACTING DNA SEQUENCES. The *cis*-acting DNA sequences are named "*cis*" because they affect the expression of only linked genes on the <u>same</u> chromosome. The *cis*-acting DNA sequences act as binding sites for various *trans*-acting proteins. There are a number of *cis*-acting DNA sequences which include the following:

1. **Core promoter sequence.** The core promoter sequence (e.g., **TATA box sequence**) is usually located **near the gene** (close to the **initiation site** where transcription actually begins) and **upstream of the gene**. The core promoter is the site where RNA polymerase II **and** TFIIs assemble to form the transcription-initiation (TI) complex so that a gene may be transcribed into an RNA transcript. However, the TI complex will produce only a **basal level of transcription** or **constitutive expression**.

2. **Proximal promoter region sequence.** The proximal promoter region sequence (e.g., **GC box sequence**) located immediately **upstream of the core promoter sequence**.

3. **Enhancer sequences.** The enhancer sequences are usually located **far away from the gene** and either **upstream or downstream of the gene**. The enhancer sequences increase the basal level of transcription or constitutive expression produced by the TI complex.

4. **Silencer sequences.** The silencer sequences can be located **near the core promoter sequence, upstream of the core promoter sequence,** or **within introns**. The silencer sequences decrease transcription levels.

5. **Insulator sequences (boundary elements).** The insulator sequences are regions of DNA that block (or insulate) the influence of enhancer sequences or silencer sequences.

6. **Response element sequences.** The response element sequences are a short distance **upstream of the core promoter sequence.** The response element sequences modulate transcription levels in response to external stimuli such as cAMP, serum growth factor, interferon-γ, heavy metals, phorbol esters, heat shock, or steroid hormones. There are a number of response element sequences which include the following:
   a. cAMP response element (CRE)
   b. Serum growth factor response element (SRE)
   c. Interferon-γ response element (IRE)
   d. Heavy metal response element (HMRE)
   e. Phorbol ester response element (PRE)
   f. Heat shock response element (HSRE)
   g. Glucocorticoid response element (GRE)

B. ***TRANS*-ACTING PROTEINS.** The *trans*-acting proteins are named "trans" because they effect the expression of genes on <u>other</u> chromosomes and migrate to their site of action. There are two types of *trans*-acting proteins called **transcription factors** and **gene regulatory proteins.** The *trans*-acting proteins bind to *cis*-acting DNA sequences.
   1. **Transcription factors.** The general transcription factors (TFIIA, TFIIB, TFII D TFIIE, TFIIF, and TFIIH) along with **RNA polymerase II** form the TI complex.
   2. **Gene regulatory proteins.** The gene regulatory proteins bind to specific enhancer sequences, silencer sequences, or insulator sequences and promote the production of **specialized proteins** within a cell (e.g., hepatocytes produce Factor VIII and the pancreatic beta cells produce insulin).
   3. **Other *trans*-acting factors.**
      a. **CREB (<u>c</u>AMP <u>r</u>esponse <u>e</u>lement <u>b</u>inding protein)** binds to CRE in response to elevated cAMP levels in the cell caused by a protein hormone binding to a G protein–linked receptor and thereby induces gene expression.
      b. **Serum response factor** binds to SRE in response to serum growth factor and thereby induces gene expression.
      c. **Stat-1** binds to IRE in response to interferon-γ and thereby induces gene expression.
      d. **Mep-1** binds to HMRE in response to heavy metals and thereby induces gene expression.
      e. **AP1** binds to PRE in response to phorbol esters and thereby induces gene expression.
      f. **hsp70** binds to HSE in response to heat shock and thereby induces gene expression.
      g. **Steroid hormone receptor** binds to GRE in response to steroid hormones and thereby induces gene expression.

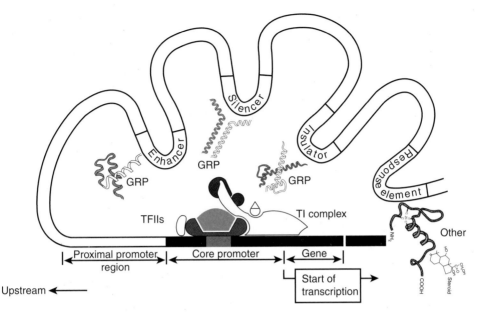

● **Figure 7-1 Mechanisms of Gene Expression.** The *cis*-acting DNA sequences include the core promoter sequence, proximal promoter region sequence, enhancer sequences, silencer sequences, insulator sequences, and response element sequences. These *cis*-acting DNA sequences act as binding sites for various *trans*-acting proteins. The *trans*-acting proteins include the general transcription factors (TFIIs), gene regulatory proteins, and other *trans*-acting proteins. The binding of the *cis*-acting DNA sequences and the *trans*-acting proteins modulate the activity of the transcription-initiation (TI) complex. DNA looping allows *trans*-acting proteins that are bound at distant sites to interact with the TI complex. GRP = gene regulatory protein; TFIIs = general transcription factors for RNA polymerase II; TI = transcription-initiation; TATA = TATA box.

Ⓘ ## The Structure of DNA-Binding Proteins. Transcription factors and gene regulatory proteins have the capability of binding to DNA. This binding capability is based on the interaction of **amino acids** of the protein with **nucleotides** of the DNA. The structure of DNA-binding proteins falls into four categories as indicated below.

A. HOMEODOMAIN PROTEINS (Figure 7-2).

The homeodomain proteins consist of three alpha helices (helix 1, 2, and 3) where helix 2 and 3 are arranged in a conspicuous **helix-turn-helix motif**. The homeodomain proteins contain a **60 amino acid** long region within helix 3 (called a **homeodomain**) that binds specifically to DNA segments. The diagram shows the three-dimensional structure of the **PIT-1 homeodomain protein (<u>pituitary</u> specific factor-<u>1</u> or GHF-1)** which is coded for by the *PIT-1* gene (also called *POU1F1* gene) on chromosome 3p11.2. The 60 amino acid homeodomain of the PIT-l protein is coded for by a 180 base pair sequence called the **homeobox sequence.** PIT-1 protein binding at the

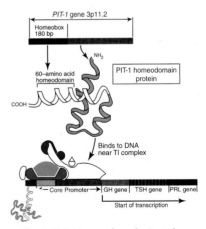

● **Figure 7-2 Homeodomain Protein.**

TI complex is required for transcription of the *GH* gene on chromosome 17q22, *TSH* gene on chromosome 1p13, and the *PRL* gene on chromosome 6p22.2. A mutation in the *PIT-1* gene will result in the combined deficiency of growth hormone (GH), thyroid stimulating hormone (TSH), and PRL (prolactin) causing **pituitary dwarfism.**

B. **LEUCINE ZIPPER PROTEINS (Figure 7-3).**
The leucine zipper proteins consist of an alpha helix that contains a region in which every seventh amino acid is leucine which has the effect of lining up all the leucine residues on one side of the alpha helix. The leucine residues allow for **dimerization** of two leucine zipper proteins to occur and form a Y-shaped dimer. Dimerization may occur between two of the same proteins (**homodimer**; e.g., JUN-JUN) or two different proteins (**heterodimer**; e.g., FOS-JUN). The leucine zipper proteins contain a **20 amino acid** long region that binds specifically to DNA segments. The diagram shows the three-dimensional structure of a leucine zipper protein (JUN) forming a leucine zipper homodimer (JUN-JUN). L: leucine. Specific examples of leucine zipper proteins are

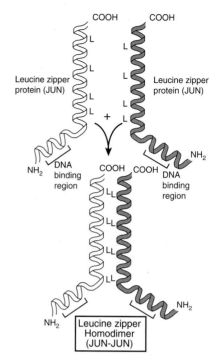

● **Figure 7-3 Leucine Zipper Protein.**

1. **C/EBP (CCAAT/enhancer binding protein)** which regulates the *ALB* gene on chromosome 4q13.3 which encodes for albumin and the *SERPINA1* gene on chromosome 14q32.1 which encodes for α1-antitrypsin (or serpin peptidase inhibitor clade A member 1).

2. **CREB (cyclic AMP response element binding protein)** which regulates the *SST* gene on chromosome 3q28 which encodes for somatostatin and the *PENK* gene on chromosome 8q23 which encodes for proenkephalin.

3. **FOS protein (Finkel osteogenic sarcoma virus)** which regulates various cell cycle genes. The FOS protein is a product of the *FOS* gene (a proto-oncogene) on chromosome 14q24.3.

4. **JUN protein** which regulates various cell cycle genes. The JUN protein is a product of the *JUN* gene (a proto-oncogene) on chromosome 1p32.

C. **HELIX-LOOP-HELIX PROTEIN (HLH; Figure 7-4).** The HLH proteins consist of a short alpha helix connected by a loop to a longer alpha helix. The loop allows for **dimerization** of two HLH proteins to occur and form a Y-shaped dimer. Dimerization may occur between two of the same proteins (**homodimers**) or two different proteins (**heterodimers**). The diagram shows the three-dimensional structure of an HLH protein forming an HLH homodimer. Specific examples of HLH proteins are

1. **MyoD protein** which regulates various genes involved in muscle development.
2. **MYC protein** which regulates various genes involved in the cell cycle. The MYC protein is encoded by the *MYC* gene (a **proto-oncogene**; v-myc <u>my</u>elo<u>c</u>ytomatosis viral oncogene homolog) on chromosome 8q24.

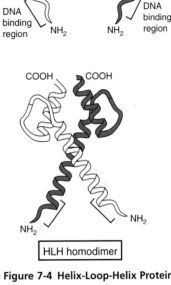

● **Figure 7-4 Helix-Loop-Helix Protein.**

D. **ZINC FINGER PROTEINS (Figure 7-5).** The zinc finger proteins consist of one alpha helix with a **zinc (Zn)** atom bound to four **cysteine** amino acids. The zinc finger proteins contain both a **hormone-binding region** and a **70 amino acid** long region near the zinc atom that binds specifically to DNA segments. The diagram shows the three-dimensional structure of a specific zinc finger protein (i.e., the glucocorticoid receptor) which behaves as a gene regulatory protein. The glucocorticoid receptor has a DNA-binding region and a steroid hormone-binding region. In the presence of

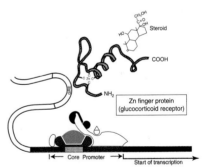

● **Figure 7-5 Zinc Finger Protein.**

glucocorticoid hormone, the glucocorticoid receptor will bind to a gene regulatory sequence known as the GRE which loops to interact with the TI complex and allows the start of gene transcription. Specific examples of zinc finger proteins are

1. **Glucocorticoid receptor**
2. **Estrogen receptor**
3. **Progesterone receptor**
4. **Thyroid hormone receptor**
5. **Retinoic acid receptor**
6. **Vitamin D3 receptor**

IV Other Mechanisms of Gene Expression

A. MICRO RNA (miRNA; Figure 7-6)

1. The miRNA genes are first transcribed into a ~70-bp RNA precursor which contains an inverted repeat. This permits double-stranded hairpin RNA formation.

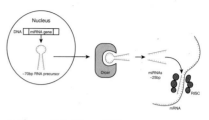

2. This ~70-bp RNA precursor is cleaved by a dsRNA-specific endonuclease called **Dicer** which produces ~25-bp RNA product called **small interfering RNA (siRNA)** or **microRNA (miRNA)**.

● Figure 7-6 Micro RNA.

3. The double-stranded miRNA unwinds to form a single-stranded miRNA which then hunts for a matching sequence on some mRNA encoding for some protein.

4. When the miRNA binds to the mRNA, an **RNA-induced silencing complex** is formed which either cleaves the mRNA or physically blocks translation. In either case, the expression of the gene that encoded the mRNA is blocked. Therefore, miRNAs seem to be very potent blockers of gene expression.

B. ANTISENSE RNA (Figure 7-7)

1. The antisense RNA genes encode for **antisense RNA** that binds to mRNA and physically blocks translation.

2. During protein synthesis, the DNA template strand is transcribed into mRNA (or **"sense"** RNA) from which a protein is translated.

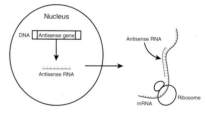

3. The DNA nontemplate strand is normally not transcribed. However, there are ~1600 genes in which the DNA nontemplate strand is also transcribed, thereby producing "antisense" RNA.

● Figure 7-7 Antisense RNA.

4. The antisense RNA then hunts for a matching sequence on the mRNA (or sense RNA) encoding for some protein.

5. When the antisense RNA binds to the sense RNA, the expression of the gene that encoded the sense RNA (or mRNA) is blocked. Therefore, antisense RNAs seem to be very potent blockers of gene expression.

C. RIBOSWITCH RNA (Figure 7-8)

1. The riboswitch genes encode for **riboswitch RNA** which binds to a target molecule, changes shape, and then switches on protein synthesis.

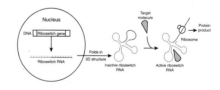

2. Riboswitch RNA folds into a complex three-dimensional shape where one portion recognizes a target molecule and the other portion contains a protein-coding RNA sequence.

● Figure 7-8 Riboswitch RNA.

3. When the riboswitch RNA binds to the target molecule, the "switch" is turned on and the protein-coding RNA sequence is translated into a protein product.

4. Note that a protein product is only formed if the riboswitch RNA binds to the target molecule.

D. ALTERNATIVE PROMOTERS AND ALTERNATIVE INTERNAL PROMOTERS

1. **Alternative promoters.** Alternative promoters start transcription from alternative versions of the first exon, which is then spliced into a common set of

downstream exons which produces an **isoform of the same molecular weight.** There are several human genes that have two or more **alternative promoters** which can result in the expression of a protein isomer.

2. **Alternative internal promoters.** Alternative internal promoters start transcription from different exons located within the gene which produces a **truncated protein with a different molecular weight.**

E. **RNA-BINDING PROTEINS.** There are a number of RNA-binding proteins that bind specifically to the **3′ UTR** (untranslated region) of mRNA and seem to be potent blockers of gene expression.

F. **ALTERNATIVE RNA SPLICING**
   1. **RNA splicing** is a process whereby all **introns (noncoding regions; intervening sequences)** are removed from the RNA transcript and all **exons (coding regions; expression sequences)** are joined together within the RNA transcript.
   2. RNA splicing is carried out by a large RNA–protein complex called the **spliceosome** which consists of **five types of small nuclear RNA** and **>50 different proteins.**
   3. Alternative RNA splicing is a process whereby different exon combinations are represented in the RNA transcript producing protein **isoforms.**

G. **X CHROMOSOME INACTIVATION**
   1. X chromosome inactivation is a process whereby either the **maternal X chromosome (X^M)** or **paternal X chromosome (X^P)** is inactivated resulting in a heterochromatin structures called the **Barr body** which is located along the inside of the nuclear envelope in female cells. This inactivation process overcomes the sex difference in **X gene dosage.**
   2. Males have one X chromosome and are therefore **constitutively hemizygous,** but females have two X chromosomes. Gene dosage is important because many X-linked proteins interact with autosomal proteins in a variety of metabolic and developmental pathways, so there needs to be a tight regulation in the amount of protein for key dosage-sensitive genes. X chromosome inactivation makes females **functionally hemizygous.**
   3. X chromosome inactivation begins early in embryological development at about the **late blastula stage.**
   4. Whether the X^M or the X^P becomes inactivated is a **random and irreversible event.** However, once a progenitor cell inactivates the X^M, for example, all the daughter cells within that cell lineage will also inactivate the X^M (the same is true for the X^P). This is called **clonal selection** and means that **all females are mosaics** comprising mixtures of cells in which either the X^M or X^P is inactivated.
   5. X chromosome inactivation does not inactivate all the genes; **≈20% of the total genes** on the X chromosome escape inactivation. These ≈20% inactivated genes include those genes that have a functional homolog on the Y chromosome (gene dosage is not affected in this case) or those genes where gene dosage is not important.
   6. The mechanism of X chromosome inactivation involves
      a. **Xic (X-inactivation center)** is a *cis*-acting DNA sequence located on the X chromosome (Xq13) which controls the **initiation and propagation of inactivation.**
      b. **Xce (X-controlling element)** is a *cis*-acting DNA sequence located on the X chromosome which affects the choice of whether X^M or X^P is inactivated.
      c. *XIST* gene (**X-inactive specific transcript**) encodes for a **17-kb RNA** that is the primary signal for **spreading the inactivation** along the X chromosome.

H. **MATERNAL MRNA**
   1. In the adult, genes are regulated at the **level of transcription-initiation.**
   2. In the early embryo, genes are regulated at the **level of translation.**

3. Immediately after fertilization of the secondary oocyte by the sperm, protein synthesis is specified by **maternal mRNAs** present within the oocyte cytoplasm.
4. These maternal mRNAs are stored in the oocyte cytoplasm in an inactive form due to **shortened poly A-tails.**
5. At fertilization, the stored inactive maternal mRNAs are activated by **polyadenylation** which restores the poly-A tail to its normal length.
6. This situation remains until the four or eight cell stage when transcription from the genome of zygote (called **zygotic transcription**) begins.

(V) The *Lac* Operon (Figure 7-9).

An operon is a set of genes adjacent to one another in the genome that are transcribed from a single promoter as one long mRNA. The *lac* operon involved in **lactose metabolism** is classic in the annals of molecular biology because the details of gene regulation were first discovered using the *lac* operon in *Escherichia coli* bacteria. Upstream of the *lac* operon lies the **lac operator, lac promoter, lac I gene, lac I promoter,** and the **CAP-binding site.** The diagram shows the four culture conditions involved in the *lac* operon.

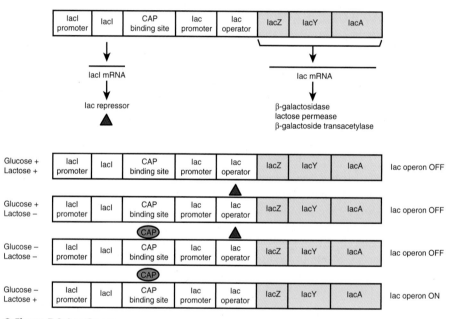

● Figure 7-9 Lac Operon.

A. The *lac* operon consists of three genes positioned in sequence:
1. *lac* Z gene: encodes **β-galactosidase** which splits (hydrolyzes) lactose into glucose and galactose.
2. *lac* Y gene: encodes **lactose permease** which pumps lactose into the cell.
3. *lac* A gene: encodes **β-galactoside transacetylase** which also splits (hydrolyzes) lactose into glucose and galactose.

B. The *lac* I gene lies upstream of the *lac* operon and is expressed separately using its own *lac* I promoter. The lac I gene encodes for a protein called the *lac* **repressor** which blocks the transcription of *lac* Z, *lac* Y, and *lac* A genes of the *lac* operon.

C. **CAP (catabolite activator protein; inducer)** is a gene regulatory protein that binds to a *cis*-acting DNA sequence (called the **CAP binding site**) upstream of the lac promoter when cAMP levels are high (↑ cAMP) and increases the transcription of *lac* Z, *lac* Y, and *lac* A genes of the *lac* operon.

D. Consequently, the *lac* operon is under the control of the *lac* repressor and CAP (inducer). This is highlighted by the response of *E. coli* to four culture conditions as indicated below:

1. **Glucose⁺ and lactose⁺ culture medium → *lac* operon OFF.** When *E. coli* is cultured in glucose⁺ and lactose⁺ culture medium, there is glucose available for metabolism. Therefore, the *lac* operon is switched off because the **lac repressor is not bound** to the lac operator and **CAP is not bound** to the CAP binding site due to ↓ **cAMP levels.**

2. **Glucose⁺ and lactose⁻ culture medium → *lac* operon OFF.** When *E. coli* is cultured in glucose⁺ and lactose⁻ culture medium, there is glucose available for metabolism. Therefore, the *lac* operon is switched off because the **lac repressor is bound** to the *lac* operator and **CAP is not bound** to the CAP binding site due to ↓ **cAMP levels.**

3. **Glucose⁻ and lactose⁻ culture medium → *lac* operon OFF.** When *E. coli* is cultured in glucose⁻ and lactose⁻ culture medium, there is no glucose available for metabolism. Therefore, the *lac* operon is switched off because the **lac repressor is bound** to the *lac* operator and **CAP is bound** to the CAP binding site due to ↑ **cAMP levels.**

4. **Glucose⁻ and lactose⁺ culture medium → *lac* operon ON.** When *E. coli* is cultured in glucose⁻ and lactose⁺ culture medium, there is no glucose available for metabolism. Therefore, the *lac* operon is switched on because the **lac repressor is not bound** to the *lac* operator and **CAP is bound** to the CAP binding site due to ↑ **cAMP levels.**

VI **The *trp* Operon (Figure 7-10).** An operon is a set of genes adjacent to one another in the genome that are transcribed from a single promoter as one long mRNA. The *trp* operon involved in **tryptophan biosynthesis** is classic in the annals of molecular biology because the details of gene regulation were first discovered using the *trp* operon in *E. coli* bacteria. Upstream of the *trp* operon lies the **trp operator, trp promoter, trp repressor gene,** and **trp repressor promoter.** The diagram shows the two culture conditions involved in the *trp* operon.

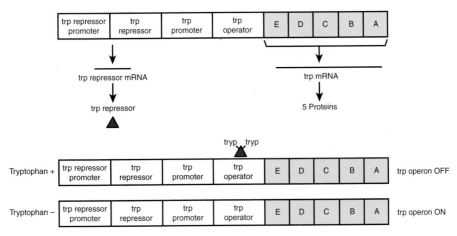

● Figure 7-10 trp Operon.

A. The *trp* operon consists of five genes positioned in sequence all of which encode for proteins that are involved in tryptophan biosynthesis.

B. The *trp* **repressor gene** lies upstream of the *trp* operon and is expressed separately using its own *trp* **repressor promoter.** The *trp* repressor gene encodes for a protein called the *trp* **repressor** which blocks the transcription of the five genes of the *trp* operon.

C. Consequently, the *trp* operon is under the control of the *trp* repressor. This is highlighted by the response of *E. coli* to two culture conditions as indicated below:

1. **Tryptophan$^+$ culture medium → *trp* operon OFF.** When *E. coli* is cultured in tryptophan$^+$ culture medium, there is tryptophan available for metabolism. Therefore, the *trp* operon is switched off because the *trp* **repressor is bound** to the *trp* operator when two molecules of tryptophan attached to the *trp* repressor and activate it.

2. **Tryptophan$^-$ culture medium → *trp* operon ON.** When *E. coli* is cultured in tryptophan$^-$ culture medium, there is no tryptophan available for metabolism. Therefore, the *trp* operon is switched on because the *trp* **repressor is not bound** to the *trp* operator because there is no tryptophan available to activate the *trp* repressor.

Chapter 8

Mutations of the DNA Sequence

I. General Features

A. The size of the human nuclear genome places huge demands on DNA polymerase to faithfully replicate the precise DNA sequence code every time a cell undergoes mitosis such that the average nucleotide diversity has been calculated. The **average nucleotide diversity = 0.08%** (i.e., 1 out of 1250 nucleotides differs on average between allelic sequences).

B. BASE SUBSTITUTIONS are the most common type of mutation and are divided into two types:
   1. Transitions involve the substitution of a purine with a purine (A ↔ G) or a pyrimidine with a pyrimidine (C ↔ T).
   2. Transversions involve the substitution of a purine with a pyrimidine (A ↔ C or T) or a pyrimidine with a purine (C ↔ A or G).

C. Mutations that occur in the ≈2% of the human nuclear genome consisting of coding DNA will clearly have the most clinical consequence. Mutations that occur in the coding DNA are grouped into two classes:
   1. Silent (synonymous) mutations where the sequence of the gene product is not changed.
   2. Non-silent (nonsynonymous) mutations where the sequence of the gene product is changed.

II. Silent (Synonymous) Mutations.

Silent mutations are mutations where a change in nucleotides alters the codon but no phenotypic change is observed in the individual. Silent mutations produce **functional proteins** and accumulate in the genome where they are called **single nucleotide polymorphisms**. A **polymorphism** is a DNA variation that is so common in the population that it <u>cannot</u> be explained by a recurring mutation. Silent mutations may occur in

A. SPACER DNA (Figure 8-1). A mutation in spacer DNA will not alter any genes or proteins.

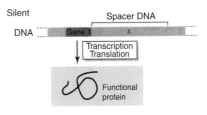

● **Figure 8-1 Silent Mutation: Spacer DNA.**

B. INTRONS (Figure 8-2). A mutation in an intron will not alter a protein because introns are spliced out as mRNA is made.

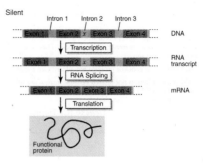

● Figure 8-2 Silent Mutation: Introns.

C. THIRD NUCLEOTIDE OF THE CODON (Figure 8-3). A mutation in the third nucleotide of the codon will not alter the protein because one amino acid has several codons. The third nucleotide can often be mutated without changing the amino acid for which it codes. This is called **third nucleotide (base) redundancy.**

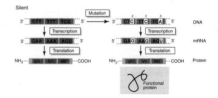

● Figure 8-3 Silent Mutation: Third Nucleotide.

III Non-Silent (Nonsynonymous) Mutations

A. MISSENSE MUTATIONS (Figure 8-4). Missense mutations are **point mutations** where a change in a single nucleotide alters the codon so that **one amino acid in a protein is replaced with another amino acid.** Missense mutations produce **proteins with a compensated function** if the mutation occurs at an active or catalytic site of the protein or alters the three dimensional structure of the protein. Missense mutations are divided into two categories:

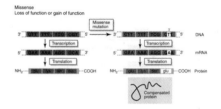

● Figure 8-4 Missense Mutation: Loss or Gain of Function.

1. **Conservative substitutions** occur when the amino acid is replaced with another amino acid that is chemically similar. The effect of such a replacement is often minimal on protein function.
2. **Nonconservative substitutions** occur when the amino acid is replaced with another amino acid that is chemically dissimilar.

B. NONSENSE MUTATIONS (Figure 8-5). Nonsense mutations are **point mutations** where a change in a single nucleotide alters the codon so that a **premature STOP codon is formed.** Nonsense mutations produce **unstable mRNAs** which are rapidly degraded or **nonfunctional (truncated) proteins.**

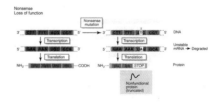

● Figure 8-5 Nonsense Mutation: Loss of Function.

C. FRAMESHIFT MUTATIONS (Figure 8-6).

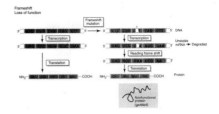

Frameshift mutations are **point mutations** where either a deletion or insertion of nucleotides (<u>not</u> a multiple of three) alters the codon so that a **premature STOP codon is formed** or the **reading frame is shifted.** Frameshift mutations produce **either unstable mRNAs** which are rapidly degraded or nonfunctional ("garbled") proteins because all of the amino acids after the deletion or insertion

● **Figure 8-6 Frameshift Mutation: Loss of Function.**

are changed, respectively. **In-frame mutations** are point mutations where either a deletion or insertion of nucleotides (a multiple of three) alters the codon but does <u>not</u> shift the reading frame. In-frame mutations produce **compensated proteins**. Clinical examples of frameshift and in-frame mutations are Duchenne muscular dystrophy (DMD) and Becker muscular dystrophy (BMD).

1. **Duchenne muscular dystrophy**
   a. DMD is an X-linked recessive genetic disorder caused by various mutations in the *DMD* gene on **chromosome Xp21.2** for **dystrophin** which anchors the cytoskeleton (actin) of skeletal muscle cells to the extracellular matrix via a transmembrane protein (**α-dystrophin and β-dystrophin**), thereby stabilizing the cell membrane. The *DMD* gene is the largest known human gene.
   b. DMD is caused by small deletion, large deletion, deletion of the entire gene, insertion, duplication of one of more exons, or single-based change mutations. The deletion or insertion of nucleotides (not a multiple of three) results in a **frameshift mutation.** These mutations result in either the **absence of dystrophin protein or a nonfunctional ("garbled") dystrophin protein** which causes severe clinical features (more severe than BMD).
   c. **Serum creatine phosphokinase (CK) measurement.** The measurement of serum CK is one of the diagnostic tests for DMD ([serum CK] = >10 times normal is diagnostic).
   d. **Skeletal muscle biopsy.** A skeletal muscle biopsy shows histological signs of fiber size variation, foci of necrosis and regeneration, hyalinization, and deposition of fat and connective tissue. Immunohistochemistry shows almost complete absence of the dystrophin protein.
   e. **Clinical features include** symptoms appear in early childhood with delays in sitting and standing independently; progressive muscle weakness (proximal weakness > distal weakness) often with calf hypertrophy; progressive muscle wasting; waddling gait; difficulty in climbing; wheelchair bound by 12 years of age; cardiomyopathy by 18 years of age; death by ≈30 years of age due to cardiac or respiratory failure.

2. **Becker muscular dystrophy**
   a. BMD is an X-linked recessive genetic disorder caused by various mutations in the *DMD* gene on **chromosome Xp21.2** for **dystrophin** which anchors the cytoskeleton (actin) of skeletal muscle cells to the extracellular matrix via a transmembrane protein (**α-dystrophin and β-dystrophin**) thereby stabilizing the cell membrane.
   b. BMD is caused by the deletion or insertion of nucleotides (a multiple of three) which results in an **in-frame mutation.** The in-frame mutation results in a **compensated dystrophin protein** which causes less severe clinical features compared with DMD.

D. RNA SPLICING MUTATIONS (Figure 8-7).

RNA splicing mutations are mutations where a change in nucleotides at the 5′-end or 3′-end of an intron alters the codon so that a **splice site in the RNA transcript is changed** which results either in **intron retention** (due to complete failure in splicing) or **exon skipping**. Intron retention generally results in a mRNA that is unable to exit the nucleus to make contact with the translational machinery and therefore **no protein** is produced. Exon skipping may re-

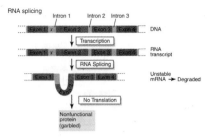

● **Figure 8-7 RNA Splicing Mutation.**

sult in a frameshift mutation where a premature **STOP codon is formed** or the **reading frame is shifted**. Frameshift mutations produce either **unstable mRNAs** which are rapidly degraded or **nonfunctional ("garbled") proteins** because all of the amino acids after the deletion or insertion are changed, respectively.

E. TRANSPOSON MUTATIONS (Figure 8-8).

Transposon mutations are mutations where a transposon alters the codon so that a gene is disrupted. Transposable element mutations produce **no protein** at all because the gene is completely disrupted. Transposition is a fairly common event in the human genome. However, in reality, it is very rare that transposition disrupts a gene.

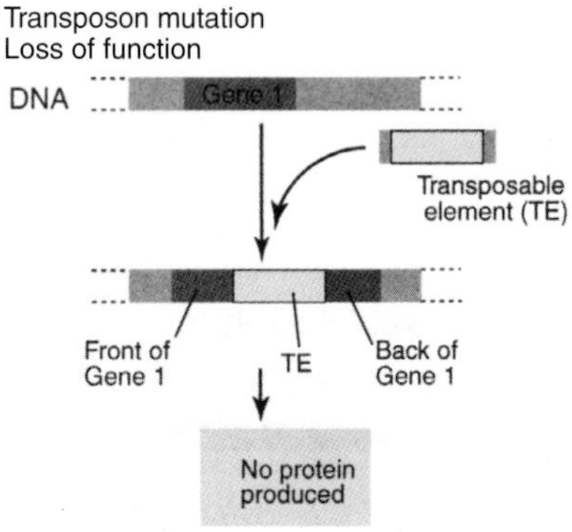

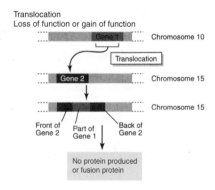

● **Figure 8-8 Transposon Mutation: Loss of Function.**

F. TRANSLOCATION MUTATIONS (Figure 8-9).

Translocation mutations are mutations where a **section of a gene is moved** from its original location to another location either on the same or different chromosome. Translocations result from breakage and exchange of segments between chromosomes. Translocation mutations produce either **no protein** or **fusion proteins with a novel function**. The following are clinical examples caused by translocations.

1. Robertsonian translocation (RT)

   a.   An RT is caused by translocations between the long arms (q) of acrocentric (satellite) chromosomes where

● **Figure 8-9 Translocation Mutation: Loss or Gain of Function.**

the breakpoint is near the centromere. The short arms (p) of these chromosomes are generally lost.

   b.   Carriers of an RT are **clinically normal** because the short arms, which are lost, contain only inert DNA and some rRNA (ribosomal RNA) genes which occur in multiple copies on other chromosomes.

   c.   One of the most common translocations found in humans is the **RT t(14q21q)**.

   d.   The clinical issue in the RT t(14q21q) occurs when the carriers produce gametes by meiosis and reproduce. Depending on how the chromosomes segregate during meiosis, conception can produce offspring with translocation trisomy 21 (live birth), translocation trisomy 14 (early miscarriage), monosomy 14 or 21 (early miscarriage), a normal chromosome complement (live birth), or a t(14q21q) carrier (live birth).

    e.   A couple where one member is a t(14q21q) carrier may have a baby with translocation trisomy 21 (Down syndrome) or recurrent miscarriages.

2. Acute promyelocytic leukemia (APL) t(15;17)(q22;q21)

    a.   APL t(15;17)(q22;q21) is caused by a reciprocal translocation between chromosomes 15 and 17 with breakpoints at bands q22 and q21, respectively.

    b.   This results in a fusion of the **promyelocyte gene (*PML* gene)** on 15q22 with the **retinoic acid receptor gene (*RARα* gene)** on 17q21, thereby forming the *PML/RARα* oncogene.

    c.   The **PML/RARα oncoprotein** (a transcription factor) blocks the differentiation of promyelocytes to mature granulocytes such that there is continued proliferation of promyelocytes.

    d.   **Clinical features include** pancytopenia (i.e., anemia, neutropenia, and thrombocytopenia), including weakness and easy fatigue, infections of variable severity, and/or hemorrhagic findings (e.g., gingival bleeding, ecchymoses, epistaxis, or menorrhagia), and bleeding secondary to disseminated intravascular coagulation. A rapid cytogenetic diagnosis of this leukemia is essential for patient management because these patients are at an extremely high risk for stroke.

3. Chronic myeloid leukemia (CML) t(9;22)(q34;q11.2)

    a.   CML t(9;22)(q34;q11.2) is caused by a reciprocal translocation between chromosomes 9 and 22 with breakpoints at q34 and q11.2, respectively. The resulting derivative chromosome 22 (der22) is referred to as the **Philadelphia chromosome.**

    b.   This results in a fusion of the *ABL* **gene** on 9q34 with the *BCR* **gene** on 22q11.1, thereby forming the *ABL/BCR* **oncogene.**

    c.   The **ABL/BCR oncoprotein** (a tyrosine kinase) has enhanced tyrosine kinase activity that transforms hematopoietic precursor cells.

    d.   **Clinical features include** systemic symptoms (e.g., fatigue, malaise, weight loss, excessive sweating), abdominal fullness, bleeding episodes due to platelet dysfunction, abdominal pain may include left upper quadrant pain, early satiety due to the enlarged spleen, tenderness over the lower sternum due to an expanding bone marrow, and the uncontrolled production of maturing granulocytes, predominantly neutrophils, but also eosinophils and basophils.

G. UNSTABLE EXPANDING REPEAT MUTATIONS (DYNAMIC MUTATIONS; Figure 8-10). Dynamic mutations are mutations that involve the **insertion of a repeat sequence** either outside or inside the gene. Dynamic mutations demonstrate a **threshold length. Below a certain threshold length,** the repeat sequence is stable, does not

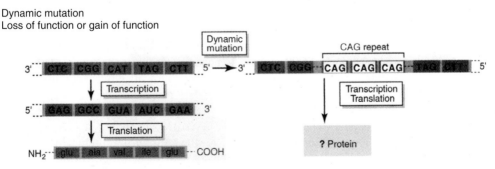

● **Figure 8-10 Dynamic Mutation: Loss or Gain of Function.**

cause disease, and is propagated to successive generations without change in length. **Above a certain threshold length**, the repeat sequence is unstable, causes disease, and is propagated to successive generations in expanding lengths. The exact mechanism by which expansion of the repeat sequences occurs is not known. One of the hallmarks of diseases caused by these mutations is **anticipation** which means the age of onset is lower and degree of severity is worsened in successive generations. Dynamic mutations are divided into two categories:

1. **Highly expanded repeats outside the gene.** In this category of dynamic mutation, various repeat sequences (e.g., CGG, CCG, GAA, CTG, CCTG, ATTCT, or CCCCGCCCCGCG) undergo very large expansions. Below threshold length expansions are ≈5–50 repeats. Above threshold length expansions are ≈100–1000 repeats. This category of dynamic mutations is characterized by the following clinical conditions.

    a. **Fragile X syndrome (Martin-Bell syndrome)**
        i. **Fragile X syndrome** is an X-linked recessive genetic disorder caused by a 200–1000+ unstable repeat sequence of $(CGG)_n$ outside the **FMR1 gene** on **chromosome X** for the **fragile X. mental retardation 1 protein (FMRP1)** which is a nucleocytoplasmic shuttling protein that binds several mRNAs found abundantly in neurons.
        ii. The 200–1000+ unstable repeat sequence of $(CGG)_n$ creates a fragile site on chromosome X which is observed when cells are cultured in a **folate-depleted** medium. The 200–1000+ unstable repeat sequence of $(CGG)_n$ has also been associated with **hypermethylation** of the **FMR1** gene so that FMRP1 is not expressed which may lead to the phenotype of fragile X.
        iii. Fragile X syndrome involves two mutation sites. **Fragile X site A** involves a 200–1000+ unstable repeat sequence of $(CGG)_n$ located in a 5′ UTR of the **FMR 1** gene on **chromosome Xq27.3**. **Fragile X site B** involves a 200+ unstable repeat sequence of $(CCG)_n$ located in a promoter region of the **FMR 1** gene on **chromosome Xq28**.
        iv. Normal **FMR1** alleles have ≈5–40 repeats. They are stably transmitted without any decrease or increase in repeat number.
        v. Premutation **FMR1** alleles have ≈59–200 repeats. They are not stably transmitted. Females with permutation **FMR1** alleles are at risk for having children with fragile X syndrome.
        vi. **Clinical features include** mental retardation (most severe in males), macroorchidism (postpubertal), speech delay, behavioral problems (e.g., hyperactivity, attention deficit), prominent forehead and jaw, joint laxity, and large dysmorphic ears. Fragile X syndrome is the second leading cause of inherited mental retardation (Down syndrome is the number one cause).

2. **Moderately expanded CAG repeats with the gene.** In this category of dynamic mutation, a CAG repeat sequence undergoes moderate expansions. Below threshold length expansions are ≈10–30 repeats. Above threshold length expansions are ≈40–200 repeats. Since CAG codes for the amino acid **glutamine**, a long tract of glutamines (polyglutamine tracts) will be inserted into the amino acid sequence of the protein and causes the protein to aggregate within certain cells. This category of dynamic mutations is characterized by the following clinical conditions.

    a. **Huntington disease (HD)**
        i. HD is an autosomal dominant genetic disorder caused by a 36 → 100+ unstable repeat sequence of $(CAG)_n$ in the coding sequence of the **HD gene** on **chromosome 4p16.3** for the **huntingtin** protein which is a widely expressed cytoplasmic protein present in neurons within the striatum, cerebral cortex, and cerebellum although its precise function is unknown.

ii. Since CAG codes for the amino acid glutamine, a long tract of glutamines (a polyglutamine tract) will be inserted into the huntingtin protein and cause protein aggregates to form within certain cells (such as implicated in other neurodegenerative disorders).

iii. Normal *HD* alleles have ≤26 repeats. They are stably transmitted without any decrease or increase in repeat number.

iv. Premutation *HD* alleles have 27–35 repeats. They are not stably transmitted. Individuals with permutation *HD* alleles are at risk for having children with HD. A child with HD inherits the expanded repeat from the father.

v. An inverse correlation exists between the number of CAG repeats and the age of HD onset: 60–100 CAG repeats = juvenile onset of HD and 36–55 CAG repeats = adult onset of HD.

vi. **Clinical features include the following:** age of onset is 35–44 years of age; mean survival time is 15–18 years after onset; a movement jerkiness most apparent at movement termination; chorea (dance-like movements); memory deficits; affective disturbances; personality changes; dementia; diffuse and marked atrophy of the neostriatum due to cell death of cholinergic neurons and GABAergic neurons within the striatum (caudate nucleus and putamen) and a relative increase in dopaminergic neuron activity; and neuronal intranuclear aggregates. The disorder is protracted and invariably fatal. In HD, homozygotes are not more severely affected by the disorder than heterozygotes, which is an exception in autosomal dominant disorders.

 IV **Loss of Function and Gain of Function Mutations.** This is another way to classify mutations that is commonly used.

A. LOSS OF FUNCTION MUTATION

1. A loss of function mutation may be caused by a missense mutation (produces a compensated protein), a nonsense mutation (produces unstable mRNAs or a non-function truncated protein), a frameshift mutation (produces unstable mRNAs or a nonfunctional garbled protein), RNA splicing mutation (produces unstable mRNAs or a nonfunctional garbled protein), transposon mutation (produces no protein), a translocation mutation (produces no protein), or a dynamic mutation. Consequently, there are many ways to cause a loss of function mutation.

2. For loss of function mutations to become clinically relevant, the individual needs to be homozygous recessive (i.e., rr); heterozygotes (i.e., Rr) are clinically normal. This is because for most genes, an individual can remain clinically normal by producing only 50% of the gene product. This is why individuals with an inborn error of metabolism disease are homozygous recessive (rr).

3. However, for a relatively few genes, an individual cannot remain clinically normal by producing only 50% of the gene product (i.e., these genes show **haploinsufficiency**). Consequently, in haploinsufficiency, the 50% reduction in gene product produces a clinically abnormal phenotype.

B. GAIN OF FUNCTION MUTATION

1. A gain of function mutation may be caused by a missense mutation (produces a compensated protein), a translocation mutation (produces a fusion protein with a novel function; PML/RARα oncoprotein or ABL/BCR oncoprotein), or a dynamic mutation. Consequently, there are not many ways to cause a gain of function mutation.

2. For gain of function mutations to become clinically relevant, the individual needs to be heterozygous (i.e., Rr). This is because the mutant allele (R) functions

abnormally despite the presence of a normal allele (r). A clinical example of a gain of function mutation involves the **Pittsburgh variant** as follows:

a. **α₁-Antitrypsin deficiency.** α_1-Antitrypsin deficiency is an autosomal recessive genetic disorder caused by a missense mutation in the *SERPINAI gene* on chromosome 14q32.1 for the <u>serpin</u> **peptidase inhibitor <u>A1</u>** (also called **α₁-antitrypsin**). In this missense mutation, methionine 358 is replaced with arginine (i.e., the **Pittsburgh variant**) which destroys the affinity for elastase. Methionine 358 at the reactive center of α_1-antitrypsin acts as a "bait" for elastase where elastase is trapped and inactivated. This protects the physiologically important **elastic fibers** present in the lung from destruction. The Pittsburgh variant results in **pulmonary emphysema** because tissue-destructive elastase is allowed to act in an uncontrolled manner in the lung. In addition, the Pittsburgh variant results in **bleeding disorder** because the Pittsburgh variant acts a potent inhibitor (gain of function) of the thrombin-fibrinogen reaction.

 Other Types of Polymorphisms. To understand polymorphisms, a number of definitions must be clear. First, a **gene** is a hereditary factor that interacts with the environment to produce a trait. Second, an **allele** is an alternative version of a gene or DNA segment. Third, a **locus** is the location of a gene or DNA segment on a chromosome (because human chromosomes are paired, humans have two alleles at each locus). Fourth, a **polymorphism** is the occurrence of two or more alleles at a specific locus in frequencies greater than can be explained by mutations alone (a polymorphism does not cause a genetic disease). Silent mutations may accumulate in the genome where they are called **single nucleotide polymorphisms**. In addition, satellite DNA, minisatellite DNA, and microsatellite DNA (all of which are tandemly repeated noncoding DNA) are prone to deletion/insertion polymorphisms, whereby the number of copies of the tandem repeat sequence varies. These are called **variable number tandem repeat (VNTR) polymorphisms**.

A. CAUSES OF VNTR POLYMORPHISMS.

VNTR polymorphisms can be caused in three ways as follows:

1. **Unequal crossover (Figure 8-11).** During Meiosis I when crossover occurs, the exchange of large segments of DNA between the maternal chromatid and paternal chromatid (i.e., nonsister chromatids) at the chiasma is an **equal exchange**, whereby the cleavage and rejoining of the chromatids occurs at the same position on the maternal chromatid and paternal chromatid. In **unequal crossover**, the cleavage and rejoining of

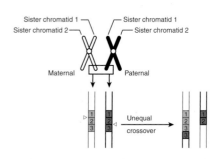

● **Figure 8-11 Unequal Crossover.**

the chromatids occurs at different positions on the maternal chromatid and paternal chromatid (i.e., nonsister chromatids) usually within a **region of tandem repeats**. This diagram shows an example of unequal crossover. A polymorphism results in the maternal chromatid having an extra repeat sequence (no. 3) obtained from the paternal chromatid (nos. 1, 2, and 3 = copies of the tandem repeat sequence).

2. **Unequal sister chromatid exchange (UESCE; Figure 8-12).** During Meiosis I when crossover occurs, the cleavage and rejoining of sister chromatids occurs at different positions on the maternal chromosome usually within a **region of tandem repeats**. Or the cleavage and rejoining of sister chromatids occurs at different positions on the paternal chromosome usually within a **region of tandem repeats**. This diagram shows an example of UESCE. A polymorphism results in one sister maternal chromatid having two repeat sequences (no. 1 and no. 3) and the other sister maternal chromatid having four repeat sequences (nos. 1, 2, 2, and 3).

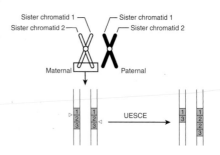

● Figure 8-12 **Unequal Sister Chromatid Exchange.**

3. **Replication slippage (Figure 8-13).** During Meiosis I when DNA replication occurs, a **region of tandem repeats** does not pair faithfully with the region of tandem repeats on its complementary strand. If the DNA loop forms on the template strand, a **forward slippage** occurs and causes a **deletion polymorphism**. If the DNA loop forms on the nascent strand, a **backward slippage** occurs and causes an **insertion polymorphism**. This diagram shows examples of replication slippage. A deletion polymorphism occurs due to forward slippage so that the newly synthesized DNA strand has no. 4 repeat sequence deleted. An insertion polymorphism occurs due to backward slippage so that the newly synthesized DNA strand has an extra no. 2 repeat sequence inserted.

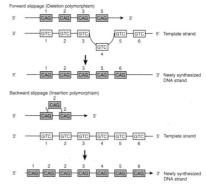

● Figure 8-13 **Replication Slippage.**

B. TYPES OF VNTR POLYMORPHISMS

1. **Large-scale VNTR polymorphisms.** Large-scale VNTR polymorphisms are typically found in **satellite DNA** which is composed of very large sized blocks (100 kb → several Mb) of tandem-repeated noncoding DNA and are formed by both unequal crossover and UESCE.

2. **Simple VNTR polymorphisms.** There are two types which include
   a. **Minisatellite DNA polymorphisms.** Minisatellite DNA polymorphisms are typically found in minisatellite DNA which is composed of moderately sized blocks (0.1 kb → 20 kb) of tandem repeated noncoding DNA and are formed by replication slippage.
   b. **Microsatellite DNA or SSR (simple sequence repeat) polymorphisms.** Microsatellite DNA or SSR polymorphisms are typically found in microsatellite DNA which is composed of small-sized blocks (1–6 bp) of tandem-repeated noncoding DNA and are formed by replication slippage.

Chapter 9

Proto-Oncogenes, Oncogenes, and Tumor-Suppressor Genes

❶ Proto-Oncogenes and Oncogenes

A. DEFINITIONS

1. A **proto-oncogene** is a normal gene that encodes a protein involved in **stimulation of the cell cycle. Because** the cell cycle can be regulated at many different points, proto-oncogenes fall into many different classes (i.e., **growth factors, receptors, signal transducers,** and transcription **factors**).

2. An **oncogene** is a mutated proto-oncogene that encodes for an **oncoprotein** involved in the **hyperstimulation of the cell cycle** leading to oncogenesis. This is because the mutations cause an increased activity of the oncoprotein (either a hyperactive oncoprotein or increased amounts of normal protein), not a loss of activity of the oncoprotein.

B. ALTERATION OF A PROTO-ONCOGENE TO AN ONCOGENE. We know now that the vast majority of human cancers are not caused by viruses. Instead, most human cancers are caused by the alteration of proto-oncogenes so that oncogenes are formed producing an oncoprotein. The mechanisms by which proto-oncogenes are altered include.

1. **Point mutation.** A point mutation (i.e., a **gain-of-function mutation**) of a proto-oncogene leads to the formation of an oncogene. A **single mutant allele** is sufficient to change the phenotype of a cell from normal to cancerous (i.e., a **dominant mutation**). This results in a hyperactive oncoprotein that hyperstimulates the cell cycle leading to oncogenesis. *Note*: proto-oncogenes only require a mutation in one allele for the cell to become oncogenic, whereas tumor-suppressor genes require a mutation in both alleles for the cell to become oncogenic.

2. **Translocation.** A translocation results from breakage and exchange of segments between chromosomes. This may result in the formation of an oncogene (also called a fusion gene or chimeric gene) which encodes for an oncoprotein (also called a fusion protein or chimeric protein). A good example is seen in chronic myeloid leukemia (CML). CML t(9;22)(q34;q11) is caused by a reciprocal translocation between chromosomes 9 and 22 with breakpoints at q34 and q11, respectively. The resulting der(22) is referred to as the **Philadelphia chromosome.** This results in a hyperactive oncoprotein that hyperstimulates the cell cycle leading to oncogenesis.

3. **Amplification.** Cancer cells may contain hundreds of extra copies of proto-oncogenes. These extra copies are found as either small paired chromatin bodies separated from the chromosomes or as insertions within normal chromosomes. This results in increased amounts of normal protein that hyperstimulates the cell cycle leading to oncogenesis.

4. **Translocation into a transcriptionally active region.** A translocation results from breakage and exchange of segments between chromosomes. This may result in the formation of an oncogene by placing a gene in a transcriptionally active region. A good example is seen in Burkitt lymphoma. **Burkitt lymphoma t(8;14)(q24;q32)** is caused by a reciprocal translocation between band q24 on chromosome 8 and band q32 on chromosome 14. This results in placing the **MYC gene** on chromosome 8q24 in close proximity to the **IGH gene** locus (i.e., an immunoglobulin gene locus) on chromosome 14q32, thereby putting the MYC gene in a transcriptionally active area in B lymphocytes (or antibody-producing plasma cells). This results in increased amounts of normal protein that hyperstimulates the cell cycle leading to oncogenesis.

C. **MECHANISM OF ACTION OF THE *RAS* GENE: A PROTO-ONCOGENE (Figure 9-1).**
    The diagram shows the *RAS* proto-oncogene and *RAS* oncogene action.

    1. The *RAS* proto-oncogene encodes a normal G-protein with GTPase activity. The G protein is attached to the cytoplasmic face of the cell membrane by a lipid called farnesyl isoprenoid. When a hormone binds to its receptor, the G protein is activated. The activated G protein binds GTP which stimulates the cell cycle. After a brief period, the activated G protein splits GTP into GDP and phosphate such that the stimulation of the cell cycle is terminated.

    2. If the *RAS* proto-oncogene undergoes a mutation, it forms the *RAS* oncogene. The *RAS* oncogene encodes an abnormal G protein (RAS oncoprotein) where a glycine is changed to a valine at position 12. The RAS oncoprotein binds GTP which stimulates the cell cycle. However, the RAS oncoprotein **cannot** split GTP into GDP and phosphate so that the stimulation of the cell cycle is never terminated.

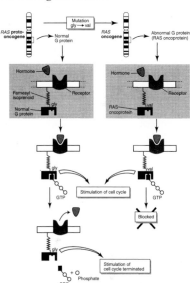

● **Figure 9-1 Action of RAS Gene.**

D. A LIST OF PROTO-ONCOGENES (Table 9-1)

TABLE 9-1			A LIST OF PROTO-ONCOGENES
Class	Protein Encoded by Proto-Oncogene	Gene	Cancer Associated with Mutations of the Proto-Oncogene
Growth factors	Platelet-derived growth factor (PDGF)	PDGFB	Astrocytoma, osteosarcoma
	Fibroblast growth factor	FGF4	Stomach carcinoma
Receptors	Epidermal growth factor receptor (EGFR)	EGFR	Squamous cell carcinoma of lung; breast, ovarian, and stomach cancers
	Receptor tyrosine kinase	RET	Multiple endocrine adenomatosis 2
	Receptor tyrosine kinase	MET	Hereditary papillary renal carcinoma, hepatocellular carcinoma
	Receptor tyrosine kinase	KIT	Gastrointestinal stromal tumors
	Receptor tyrosine kinase	ERBB2	Neuroblastoma, breast cancer
Signal transducers	Tyrosine kinase	ABL/BCR	CML t(9;22)(q34;q11)*
	Serine/threonine kinase	BRAF	Melanoma, colorectal cancer
	RAS G-proteins	HRAS KRAS NRAS	Lung, colon, and pancreas cancers
Transcription factors	Leucine zipper protein	FOS	Finkel-Biskes-Jinkins osteosarcoma
	Leucine zipper protein	JUN	Avian sarcoma 17
	Helix-loop-helix protein	N-MYC	Neuroblastoma
	Helix-loop-helix protein	L-MYC	Lung carcinoma
	Helix-loop-helix protein	MYC	Burkitt lymphoma t(8;14)(q24;q32)
	Retinoic acid receptor	PML/RARα	APL t(15;17)(q22;q12)
	Transcription factor	FUS/ERG	AML t(16;21)(p11;q22)
	Transcription factor	PBX/TCF3	Pre-B cell ALL t(1;19)(q21;p13.3)
	Transcription factor	FOXO4/MLL	ALL t(X;11)(q13;q23)
	Transcription factor	FLI1/EWSR1	Ewing sarcoma t(11;22)(q24;q12)

PDGFB = platelet-derived growth factor beta gene; FGF4 = fibroblast growth factor 4 gene; EGFR = epidermal growth factor receptor gene; RET = rearranged during transfection gene; MET = met proto-oncogene (hepatocyte growth factor receptor); KIT = v-kit Hardy-Zuckerman 4 feline sarcoma viral oncogene homolog; ERBB2 = v-erb-b2 erythroblastic leukemia viral oncogene homolog 2; ABL/BCR = Abelson murine leukemia/breakpoint cluster region oncogene; BRAF = v-raf murine sarcoma viral oncogene homolog B1; HRAS = Harvey rat sarcoma viral oncogene homolog; KRAS = Kirsten rat sarcoma 2 viral oncogene homolog; NRAS = neuroblastoma rat sarcoma viral oncogene homolog; FOS = Finkel-Binkes-Jinkins osteosarcoma; N-MYC = neuroblastoma v-myc myelocytomatosis viral oncogene homolog; MYC = v-myc myelocytomatosis viral oncogene homolog; PML/RARα = promyelocytic leukemia/retinoic acid receptor alpha; FUS/ERG = fusion (involved in t(12;16) in malignant liposarcoma)/v-ets erythroblastosis virus E26 oncogene homolog; PBX/TCF3 = pre-B-cell leukemia homeobox/transcription factor 3 (E2A immunoglobulin enhancer binding factors E12/E47); FOXO4/MLL = forkhead box O4/myeloid/lymphoid or mixed-lineage leukemia; FLI1/EWSR1 = Friend leukemia virus integration 1/Ewing sarcoma breakpoint region 1.
ALL = acute lymphoblastoid leukemia; CML = chronic myeloid leukemia; APL = acute promyelocytic leukemia; AML = acute myelogenous leukemia.

II **Tumor-Suppressor Genes.** A **tumor-suppressor gene** is a normal gene that encodes a protein involved in **suppression of the cell cycle**. Many human cancers are caused by **loss-of-function mutations** of tumor-suppressor genes. *Note*: tumor-suppressor genes require a mutation in both alleles for a cell to become oncogenic, whereas, proto-oncogenes only require a mutation in one allele for a cell to become oncogenic. Tumor-suppressor genes can be either "gatekeepers" or "caretakers."

A. GATEKEEPER TUMOR-SUPPRESSOR GENES.
These genes encode for proteins that either regulate the transition of cells through the checkpoints ("gates") of the cell cycle or promote apoptosis. This prevents oncogenesis. Loss-of-function mutations in gatekeeper tumor-suppressor genes lead to oncogenesis.

B. **CARETAKER TUMOR-SUPPRESSOR GENES.** These genes encode for proteins that either detect/repair DNA mutations or promote normal chromosomal disjunction during mitosis. This prevents oncogenesis by maintaining the integrity of the genome. Loss-of-function mutations in caretaker tumor-suppressor genes lead to oncogenesis.

C. **MECHANISM OF ACTION OF THE *RB1* GENE: A TUMOR-SUPPRESSOR GENE (RETINOBLASTOMA; Figure 9-2).** The diagram shows *RB1* tumor-suppressor gene action.

1. The *RB1* tumor-suppressor gene is located on chromosome 13q14.1 and encodes for **normal RB protein** that will bind to E2F (a gene regulatory protein) such that there will be no expression of target genes whose gene products stimulate the cell cycle. Therefore, there is suppression of the cell cycle at the G1 checkpoint.

2. A mutation of the *RB1* tumor-suppressor gene will encode an **abnormal RB protein** that cannot bind E2F (a gene regulatory protein) such that there will be expression of target genes whose gene products stimulate the cell cycle. Therefore, there is no suppression of the cell cycle at the G1 checkpoint. This leads to the formation of a **retinoblastoma** tumor.

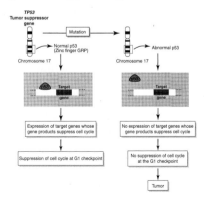

● **Figure 9-2** Action of RB1 Gene.

3. There are two types of retinoblastomas.
   a. In **hereditary retinoblastoma (RB)**, the individual inherits one mutant copy of the *RB1* gene from his parents (an inherited germline mutation). A somatic mutation of the second copy of the *RB1* gene may occur later in life within many cells of the retina leading to **multiple tumors in both eyes**.
   b. In **nonhereditary RB, the** individual does **not** inherit a mutant copy of the *RB1* gene from his parents. Instead, two subsequent somatic mutations of both copies of the *RB1* gene may occur within one cell of the retina leading to **one tumor in one eye**. This has become known as Knudson's two-hit hypothesis and serves as a model for cancers involving tumor-suppressor genes.

D. **MECHANISM OF ACTION OF THE *TP53* GENE: A TUMOR-SUPPRESSOR GENE ("GUARDIAN OF THE GENOME") (Figure 9-3).** The diagram shows *TP53* tumor-suppressor gene action.

1. The *TP53* tumor-suppressor gene is located on chromosome 17p13 and encodes for **normal p53 protein (a zinc finger gene regulatory protein)** that will cause the expression of target genes whose gene products suppress the cell cycle at G1 by inhibiting **Cdk-cyclin D** and **Cdk-cyclin E**. Therefore, there is suppression of the cell cycle at the G1 checkpoint.

2. A mutation of *TP53* tumor-suppressor gene will encode an **abnormal p53 protein** that will cause no expression of target genes whose gene products suppress the cell

● **Figure 9-3** Action of TP53 Gene.

cycle. Therefore, there is no suppression of the cell cycle at the G1 checkpoint. The *TP53* tumor-suppressor gene is the **most common target** for mutation in human cancers. The *TP53* tumor-suppressor gene plays a role in **Li-Fraumeni syndrome**.

E. A LIST OF TUMOR-SUPPRESSOR GENES (Table 9-2)

TABLE 9-2	A LIST OF TUMOR-SUPPRESSOR GENES		
Class	Protein Encoded by Tumor-Suppressor Gene	Gene	Cancer Associated with Mutations of the Tumor-Suppressor Gene
Gatekeeper	Retinoblastoma associated protein p110^{RB}	*RB1*	Retinoblastoma, carcinomas of the breast, prostate, bladder, and lung
	Tumor protein 53	*TP53*	Li-Fraumeni syndrome; most human cancers
	Neurofibromin protein	*NF1*	Neurofibromatosis type 1, Schwannoma
	Adenomatous polyposis coli protein	*APC*	Familial adenomatous polyposis coli, carcinomas of the colon
	Wilms tumor protein 2	*WT2*	Wilms tumor (most common renal malignancy of childhood)
	Von Hippel-Lindau disease tumor-suppressor protein	*VHL*	Von Hippel-Lindau disease, retinal and cerebellar hemangioblastomas
Caretaker	Breast cancer type 1 susceptibility protein	*BRCA1*	Breast and ovarian cancer
	Breast cancer type 2 susceptibility protein	*BRCA2*	Breast cancer in BOTH breasts
	DNA mismatch repair protein MLH1	*MLH1*	Hereditary nonpolyposis colon cancer
	DNA mismatch repair protein MSH2	*MSH2*	Hereditary nonpolyposis colon cancer

APC = familial <u>a</u>denomatous <u>p</u>olyposis <u>c</u>oli; *VHL* = <u>v</u>on <u>H</u>ippel-<u>L</u>indau disease; *WT* = <u>W</u>ilms <u>t</u>umor; *NF-1* = <u>n</u>euro<u>f</u>ibromatosis; *BRCA* = <u>br</u>east <u>ca</u>ncer; *RB* = <u>r</u>etino<u>b</u>lastoma; *TP53* = <u>t</u>umor <u>p</u>rotein; *MLH1* = <u>m</u>ut <u>L</u> homolog 1; *MSH2* = <u>m</u>ut <u>S</u> homolog 2.

III Hereditary Cancer Syndromes

A. HEREDITARY RETINOBLASTOMA (Figure 9-4)

1. Hereditary RB is an **autosomal dominant** genetic disorder caused by a mutation in the *RB1* gene on **chromosome 13q14.1-q14.2** for the **RB-associated protein (p110^{RB})**. More than 1000 different mutations of the *RB1* gene have been identified, which include missense, frameshift, and RNA splicing mutations which result in a premature STOP codon and a **loss-of-function mutation**.

2. RB protein binds to E2F (a gene regulatory protein) such that there will be no expression of target genes whose gene products stimulate the cell cycle at the G1 checkpoint. The RB protein belongs to the family of **tumor-suppressor genes**.

3. Hereditary RB affected individuals inherit one mutant copy of the *RB1* gene from their parents (an inherited germline mutation) followed by a somatic mutation of the second copy of the *RB1* gene later in life.

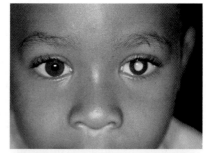

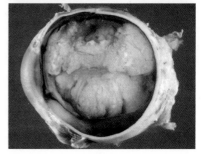

● **Figure 9-4 Hereditary Retinoblastoma.**

4. **Parents of the proband.** The proband may have an RB affected parent or an unaffected parent who has an *RB1* gene mutation. If the proband mutation is identified in either parent, then the parent is at risk of transmitting that *RB1* gene mutation to other offspring. If the proband mutation is not identified in either parent, then the proband has a *de novo RB1* gene germline mutation (90%–94% chance) or one parent is mosaic for the *RB1* gene mutation (6%–10% chance).

5. How can cancer due to tumor-suppressor genes be autosomal dominant when both copies of the gene must be inactivated for tumor formation to occur? The inherited deleterious allele is in fact transmitted in an autosomal dominant manner and most heterozygotes do develop cancer. However, while the predisposition for cancer is inherited in an **autosomal dominant manner**, changes at the cellular level require the loss of both alleles, which is a **recessive mechanism**.

6. **Clinical features:** a malignant tumor of the retina develops in children <5 years of age; whitish mass in the pupillary area behind the lens (leukokoria; the cat's eye; white eye reflex) and strabismus.

7. The top photograph shows a white pupil (leukokoria; cat's eye) in the left eye. The bottom photograph of a surgical specimen shows an eye that is almost completely filled a cream-colored intraocular retinoblastoma.

B. CLASSIC LI-FRAUMENI SYNDROME (LFS)

1. Classic LFS is an autosomal dominant genetic disorder caused by a mutation in the *TP53* gene on **chromosome 17p13.1** for the **cellular tumor protein 53** ("the **guardian of the genome**"). Mutations of the *TP53* gene have been identified which include missense (80%) and RNA splicing (20%) mutations which result in a premature STOP codon and a **loss-of-function mutation**.

2. The activation (i.e., phosphorylation) of p53 causes the transcriptional upregulation of **p21**. The binding of p21 to the Cdk2-cyclin D and Cdk2-cyclin E inhibits their action and causes downstream stoppage at the G_1 checkpoint. p53 belongs to the family of **tumor-suppressor genes**.

3. **Clinical features include** a highly penetrant cancer syndrome associated with soft-tissue sarcoma, breast cancer, leukemia, osteosarcoma, melanoma, and cancers of the colon, pancreas, adrenal cortex, and brain; 50% of the affected individuals develop cancer by 30 years of age and 90% by 70 years of age; an increased risk for developing multiple primary cancers; LFS is defined by a proband with a sarcoma diagnosed <45 years of age AND a first-degree relative <45 years of age with any cancer AND a first- or second-degree relative <45 years of age with any cancer.

C. NEUROFIBROMATOSIS TYPE 1 (NF1; VON RECKLINGHAUSEN DISEASE; Figure 9-5)

1. NF1 is a relatively common **autosomal dominant** genetic disorder caused by a mutation in the *NF1* gene on **chromosome 17q11.2** for the **neurofibromin** protein. More than 500 different mutations of the *NF1* gene have been identified which include missense, nonsense, frameshift, whole gene deletions, intragenic deletions, and RNA splicing mutations, all of which result in a **loss-of-function mutation**.

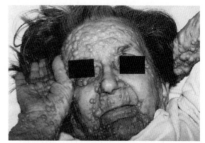

● Figure 9-5 Neurofibromatosis Type 1.

2. Neurofibromin downregulates **p21 RAS oncoprotein** so that the *NF1* gene belongs to the family of **tumor-suppressor genes** and regulates cAMP levels.

3. **Clinical features include** multiple neural tumors (called **neurofibromas** that are widely dispersed over the body and reveal proliferation of all elements of a peripheral nerve including neurites, fibroblasts, and Schwann cells of neural crest origin), numerous pigmented skin lesions (called **café au lait spots**) probably associated with melanocytes of neural crest origin, axillary and inguinal freckling, scoliosis, vertebral dysplasia, and pigmented iris hamartomas (called **Lisch nodules**).

4. The photograph shows a woman with generalized neurofibromas on the face and arms.

D. FAMILIAL ADENOMATOUS POLYPOSIS COLI (FAPC; Figure 9-6)

1. FAPC is an autosomal dominant genetic disorder caused by a mutation in the *APC* gene on **chromosome 5q21-q22** for the **adenomatous polyposis coli protein**. More than 800 different germline mutations of the *APC* gene have been identified all of which result in a **loss-of-function mutation**. The most common germline APC mutation is a **5-bp deletion** at codon 1309.

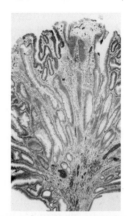

2. APC protein binds **glycogen synthase kinase 3b (GSK-3b)** which targets **β-catenin**. APC protein maintains normal apoptosis and inhibits cell proliferation through the **Wnt signal transduction pathway** so that *APC* gene belongs to the family of **tumor-suppressor genes**.

3. A majority of colorectal cancers develop slowly through a series of histopathological changes each of which has been associated with mutations of specific proto-oncogenes and tumor-suppressor genes as follows: normal epithelium → a small polyp involves mutation of the *APC* tumor-suppressor gene; small polyp → large

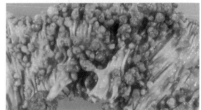

● **Figure 9-6 Familial Adenomatous Polyposis Coli.**

polyp involves mutation of *RAS* proto-oncogene; large polyp → carcinoma → metastasis involves mutation of the *DCC* tumor-suppressor gene and the *TP53* tumor-suppressor gene.

4. **Clinical features include** colorectal adenomatous polyps appear at 7–35 years of age inevitably leading to colon cancer; thousands of polyps can be observed in the colon; gastric polyps may be present; and patients are often advised to undergo prophylactic colectomy early in life to avert colon cancer.

5. The top light micrograph shows an adenomatous polyp. A polyp is a tumorous mass that extends into the lumen of the colon. Note the convoluted, irregular arrangement of the intestinal glands with the basement membrane intact. The bottom photograph shows the colon that contains thousands of adenomatous polyps.

E. BRCA1 AND BRCA2 HEREDITARY <u>BREAST</u> <u>CA</u>NCERS (Figure 9-7)

1. BRCA1 and BRCA2 hereditary breast cancers are autosomal genetic disorders caused by a mutation in either the *BRCA1* **gene** on **chromosome 17q21** for the <u>breast</u> <u>ca</u>ncer type 1 susceptibility protein or a mutation in the *BRCA2* **gene** on chromosome 13q12.3 for the **breast cancer type 2 susceptibility protein.**

2. BRCA type 1 and type 2 susceptibility proteins bind RAD51 protein which plays a role in **double-strand DNA break repair** so that *BRCA1* and *BRCA2* genes belong to the family of **tumor-suppressor genes.**

3. More than 600 different mutations of the *BRCA1* gene have been identified all of which result in a **loss-of-function mutation.**

4. More than 450 different mutations of the *BRCA2* gene have been identified all of which result in a **loss-of-function mutation.**

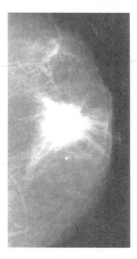

● **Figure 9-7 Mammogram of Breast Cancer.**

5. **Prevalence.** The prevalence of *BRCA1* gene mutations is 1/1000 in the general population. A population study of breast cancer found a prevalence of *BRCA1* gene mutations in only 2.4% of the cases. A predisposition to breast, ovarian, and prostate cancer may be associated with mutations in the *BRCA1* gene and *BRCA2* gene although the exact percentage of risk is not known and even appears to be variable within families.

6. **Clinical features include** early onset of breast cancer, bilateral breast cancer, family history of breast or ovarian cancer consistent with autosomal dominant inheritance, and a family history of male breast.

7. The mammogram shows a malignant mass that has the following characteristics: shape is irregular with many lobulations; margins are irregular or spiculated; density is medium-high; breast architecture may be distorted; and calcifications (not shows) are small, irregular, variable, and found within ducts (called ductal casts).

Chapter 10

The Cell Cycle

① Mitosis (Figure 10-1). Mitosis is the process by which a cell with the diploid number of chromosomes, which in humans is 46, passes on the diploid number of chromosomes to daughter cells. The term "**diploid**" is classically used to refer to a cell containing 46 chromosomes. The term "**haploid**" is classically used to refer to a cell containing 23 chromosomes. The process ensures that the diploid number of 46 chromosomes is maintained in the cells. Mitosis occurs at the end of a cell cycle. Phases of the cell cycle are as follows:

A. **G_0 (GAP) PHASE.** The G_0 phase is the resting phase of the cell. The amount of time a cell spends in G_0 is variable and depends on how actively a cell is dividing.

B. **G_1 PHASE.** The G_1 phase is the gap of time between mitosis (M phase) and DNA synthesis (S phase). The G_1 phase is the phase where **RNA, protein, and organelle synthesis** occurs. The G_1 phase lasts about **5 hours** in a typical mammalian cell with a 16-hour cell cycle.

C. **G_1 CHECKPOINT. Cdk2-cyclin D and Cdk2-cyclin E** mediate the $G_1 \rightarrow S$ phase transition at the G_1 checkpoint.

D. **S (SYNTHESIS) PHASE.** The S phase is the phase where **DNA synthesis** occurs. The S phase lasts about **7 hours** in a typical mammalian cell with a 16-hour cell cycle.

E. **G_2 PHASE.** The G_2 phase is the gap of time between DNA synthesis (S phase) and mitosis (M phase). The G_2 phase is the phase where high levels of **ATP synthesis** occur. The G_2 phase lasts about **3 hours** in a typical mammalian cell with a 16-hour cell cycle.

F. **G_2 CHECKPOINT. Cdk1-cyclin A and Cdk1-cyclin B** mediate the $G_2 \rightarrow M$ phase transition at the G_2 checkpoint.

G. **M (MITOSIS) PHASE.** The M phase is the phase where **cell division** occurs. The M phase is divided into six stages called **prophase, prometaphase, metaphase, anaphase, telophase,** and **cytokinesis.** The M phase lasts about 1 hour in a typical mammalian cell with a 16-hour cell cycle.
   1. **Prophase.** The chromatin condenses to form well-defined chromosomes. Each chromosome has been duplicated during the S phase and has a specific DNA sequence called the **centromere** that is required for proper segregation. The **centrosome complex,** which is the **microtubule-organizing center,** splits into two, and each half begins to move to opposite poles of the cell. The **mitotic spindle** (microtubules) forms between the centrosomes.
   2. **Prometaphase.** The nuclear envelope is disrupted which allows the microtubules access to the chromosomes. The nucleolus disappears. The **kinetochores** (protein complexes) assemble at each centromere on the chromosomes. Certain microtubules of the mitotic spindle bind to the kinetochores and are called **kinetochore microtubules.** Other microtubules of the mitotic spindle are now called **polar microtubules** and **astral microtubules.**

Figure 10-1 | **The Cell Cycle**

G_0 Phase
Resting phase
Cell cycle suspended

↓

G_1 Phase
Lasts 5 hours
RNA, protein, and organelle synthesis
Cdk2-cyclin D and Cdk2-cyclin E synthesis

Cdk2-cyclin D
Cdk2-cyclin E　⊕──→G_1 checkpoint

↓

S Phase
Lasts 7 hours
DNA synthesis
RNA and histone synthesis
Centrosome (MTOC) duplicates but remains together as a complex on one side of the nucleus
Methotrexate (Folex), 5-fluorouracil (Adrucil), Cytarabine (cytosine arabinoside), 6-mer-captopurine, Doxorubicin (Adriamycin), Daunorubicin (Cerubidine) are S phase specific

↓　　←——Etoposide prevents entry into G_2 phase

G_2 Phase
Lasts 3 hours
ATP synthesis
Cdk1-cyclin A and Cdk1-cyclin B synthesis
Bleomycin (Blenoxane) is G_2 phase specific

Cdk1-cyclin A
Cdk1-cyclin B　⊕──→G_2 checkpoint

↓

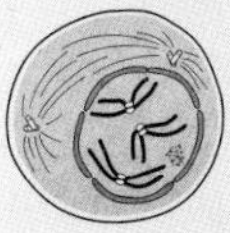

PROPHASE
Chromatin condenses to form well-defined chromosomes
Each chromosome has been duplicated during the S phase and has a specific DNA sequence called the **centromere** that is required for proper segregation
The **centrosome complex** which is the **microtubule organizing center (MTOC)** splits into two and each half begins to move to opposite poles of the cell
The **mitotic spindle** (microtubules) forms between the centrosomes

↓

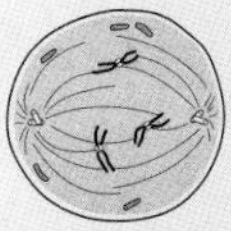

PROMETAPHASE
Nuclear envelope is disrupted which allows the microtubules access to the chromosomes
Nucleolus disappears
Kinetochores (protein complexes) assemble at each centromere on the chromosomes
Certain microtubules of the mitotic spindle bind to the kinetochores and are called **kinetochore microtubules**
Other microtubules of the mitotic spindle are now called **polar microtubules** and **astral microtubules**

↓

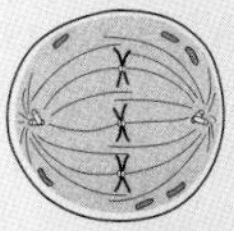

METAPHASE
Chromosomes align at the **metaphase plate**
Cells can be arrested in this stage by microtubule inhibitors (e.g., colchicine)
Cells can be isolated in this stage for **karyotype analysis**

↓

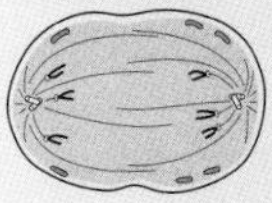

ANAPHASE
Kinetochores separate and chromosomes move to opposite poles
Kinetochore microtubules shorten and Polar microtubules lengthen

↓

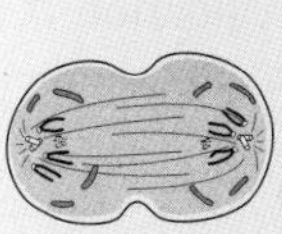

TELOPHASE
Chromosomes begin to decondense to form chromatin
Nuclear envelope re-forms
Nucleolus reappears
Kinetochore microtubules disappear
Polar microtubules continue to lengthen

↓

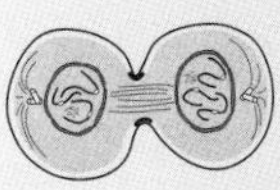

CYTOKINESIS
Cytoplasm divides by a process called **cleavage**
A **cleavage furrow** forms around the middle of the cell
A **contractile ring** consisting of actin and myosin filaments is found at the cleavage furrow

Interphase Lasts 15 hours

M Phase Last 1 hour Vinblastin (Velban), Vincristine (oncovin), Pazlitaxel (Taxol) are M phase specific

3. **Metaphase.** The chromosomes align at the metaphase plate. The cells can be arrested in this stage by microtubule inhibitors (e.g., colchicine). The cells arrested in this stage can be used for **karyotype analysis.**

4. **Anaphase.** The centromeres split, the kinetochores separate, and the chromosomes move to opposite poles. The kinetochore microtubules shorten. The polar microtubules lengthen.

5. **Telophase.** The chromosomes begin to decondense to form chromatin. The nuclear envelope re-forms. The nucleolus reappears. The kinetochore microtubules disappear. The polar microtubules continue to lengthen.

6. **Cytokinesis.** The cytoplasm divides by a process called **cleavage.** A **cleavage furrow** forms around the middle of the cell. A **contractile ring** consisting of actin and myosin filaments is found at the cleavage furrow.

Ⅱ **Control of the Cell Cycle (Figure 10-2).** The control of the cell cycle involves three main components which include

A. **CDK-CYCLIN COMPLEXES.** The two main protein families that control the cell cycle are **cyclins** and the **cyclin-dependent protein kinases (Cdks).** A cyclin is a protein that regulates the activity of Cdks and is so named because cyclins undergo a cycle of synthesis and degradation during the cell cycle. The cyclins and Cdks form complexes called **Cdk-cyclin complexes.** The ability of Cdks to phosphorylate target proteins is dependent on the particular cyclin that complex with it.

1. **Cdk2-cyclin D and Cdk2-cyclin E** mediate the $G_1 \rightarrow S$ phase transition at the G_1 checkpoint.

2. **Cdk1-cyclin A and Cdk1-cyclin B** mediate the $G_2 \rightarrow M$ phase transition at the G_2 checkpoint.

B. **CHECKPOINTS.** The checkpoints in the cell cycle are specialized signaling mechanisms that regulate and coordinate the cell response to **DNA damage** and **replication fork blockage.** When the extent of DNA damage or replication fork blockage is beyond the steady-state threshold of DNA repair pathways, a checkpoint signal is produced and a checkpoint is activated. The activation of a checkpoint slows down the cell cycle so that DNA repair may occur and/or blocked replication forks can be recovered. **This prevents DNA damage from being converted into inheritable mutations producing highly transformed, metastatic cells.**

1. **Control of the G_1 checkpoint.** There are three pathways that control the G_1 checkpoint which include

   a. Depending on the type of the DNA damage, **ATR kinase** and **ATM kinase** will activate (i.e., phosphorylate) **Chk1 kinase** or **Chk2 kinase**, respectively. The activation of Chk1 kinase or Chk2 kinase causes the inactivation of **CDC25 A phosphatase.** The inactivation of CDC25 A phosphatase causes the downstream stoppage at the G_1 checkpoint.

   b. Depending on the type of the DNA damage, **ATR kinase** and **ATM kinase** will activate (i.e., phosphorylate) **p53**, which allows p53 to disassociate from **Mdm2.** The activation of p53 causes the transcriptional upregulation of **p21.** The binding of p21 to the Cdk2-cyclin D and Cdk2-cyclin E inhibits their action and causes downstream stoppage at the G_1 checkpoint.

   c. Depending on the type of the DNA damage, **ATR kinase** and **ATM kinase** will activate (i.e., phosphorylate) **p16**, which inactivates **Cdk4/6-cyclin D** and thereby causes downstream stoppage at the G_1 checkpoint.

2. **Control of the G$_2$ checkpoint.** Depending on the type of the DNA damage, **ATR kinase** and **ATM kinase** will activate (i.e., phosphorylate) **Chk1 kinase** or **Chk2 kinase**, respectively. The activation of Chk1 kinase or Chk2 kinase causes the inactivation of **CDC25 C phosphatase**. The deactivation of CDC25 C phosphatase will cause the downstream stoppage at the G$_2$ checkpoint.

C. **INACTIVATION OF CYCLINS.** Cyclins are inactivated by **protein degradation** during **anaphase of the M phase**. The cyclin genes contain a homologous DNA sequence called a **destruction box**. A specific **recognition protein** binds to the amino acid sequence coded by the destruction box that allows **ubiquitin** (a 76 amino acid protein) to be covalently attached to lysine residues of cyclin by the enzyme **ubiquitin ligase**. This process is called **polyubiquitination**. Polyubiquitinated cyclins are rapidly degraded by proteolytic enzyme complexes called a **proteosome**. Polyubiquitination is a widely occurring process for marking many different types of proteins (cyclins are just a specific example) for rapid degradation.

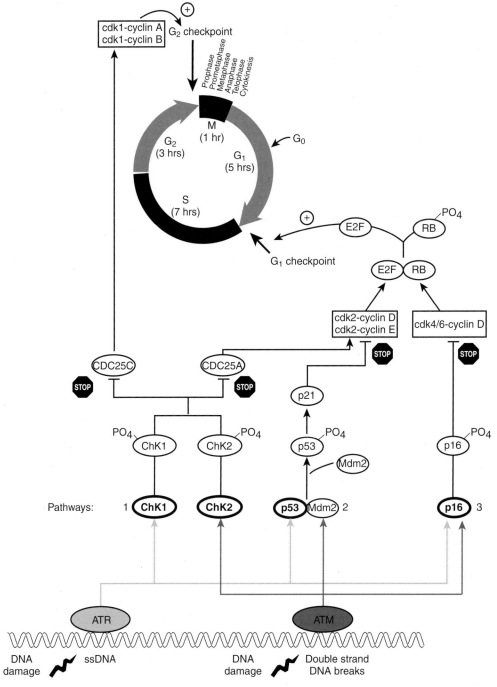

● **Figure 10-2 Diagram of the cell cycle with checkpoints and signaling mechanisms.** ATR kinase responds to the sustained presence of single-stranded DNA (ssDNA) because ssDNA is generated in virtually all types of DNA damage and replication fork blockage by activation (i.e., phosphorylation) of **Chk1 kinase, p53,** and **p16.** ATM kinase responds particularly to **double-stranded DNA breaks** by activation (i.e., phosphorylation) of **Chk2 kinase, p53,** and **p16.** The downstream pathway past the STOP sign is as follows: Cdk2-cyclinD, Cdk2-cyclinE, and Cdk4/6-cyclinD phosphorylate the E2F-RB complex which causes phosphorylated RB to disassociate from E2F. E2F is a transcription factor that causes the expression of gene products that stimulate the cell cycle. Note the location of the four stop signs. → = activation; ⊤ = inactivation.

Chapter 11

Molecular Biology of Cancer

The Development of Cancer (Oncogenesis). In general, cancer is caused by mutations of genes that regulate the **cell cycle, DNA repair,** and/or **programmed cell death (i.e., apoptosis).** A majority of cancers (so-called **sporadic cancers**) are caused by mutations of these genes in somatic cells that then divide wildly and develop into a cancer. A minority of cancers (so-called **hereditary cancers**) are predisposed by mutations of these genes in the parental germ cells that are then passed on to their children. In addition, certain cancers are linked to **environmental factors** as prime etiological importance (e.g., bladder cancer/aniline dyes, lung cancer/smoking or asbestos, liver angiosarcoma/polyvinyl chloride, skin cancer/tar, or UV irradiation). From a scientific point of view, the cause of cancer is not entirely a mystery but still remains in the theoretical arena which include the following:

A. **STANDARD THEORY (Figure 11-1).** The standard theory suggests that cancer is the result of cumulative **mutations in proto-oncogenes** (e.g., *RAS* gene) **and/or tumor-suppressor genes** (e.g., *TP53* gene) eventually producing a cancer cell. However, if cancer is caused only by mutations in these specific cell cycle genes, it is very hard to explain the appearance of the nucleus in a cancer cell. The nucleus in a cancer cells looks as if something has detonated an explosion resulting in an array of chromosomal aberrations (e.g., chromosome pieces, scrambled chromosomes, chromosomes fused together, wrong number of chromosomes, chromosomes with missing arms, or chromosome with extra segments; so-called **karyotype chaos**). The question is "Which comes first, the mutations in cell cycle genes or the chromosomal aberrations?" The photograph (left side) shows a normal human karyotype. The photograph (right side) shows an abnormal human karyotype due to a mutation involving the RAD 17 checkpoint protein which plays a role in the cell cycle. This mutation results in a re-replication of already replicated DNA and an abnormal karyotype.

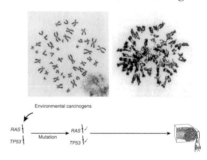

● Figure 11-1 Standard Theory.

B. **MODIFIED STANDARD THEORY (Figure 11-2).** The modified standard theory suggests that cancer is the result of a **dramatically elevated random mutation rate** caused by environmental carcinogens or malfunction in the DNA replication machinery or DNA repair machinery. The random mutations eventually hit the proto-oncogenes (e.g., *RAS* gene) and/or tumor-suppressor genes (e.g., *TP53* gene) producing a cancer cell.

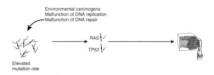

● Figure 11-2 Modified Standard Theory.

C. **EARLY INSTABILITY THEORY (Figure 11-3).**
The early instability theory suggests that cancer is the result of **disabling (either by mutation or epigenetically) of "master genes" that
are required for cell division.** No specific master genes have been identified. Therefore, each
time a cell undergoes the complex process of

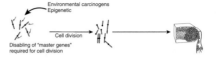

● Figure 11-3 Early Instability Theory.

cell division, some daughter cells get chromosomes fused together, the wrong number
of chromosomes, chromosomes with missing arms, or chromosome with extra segments
which will affect **gene dosage** of the proto-oncogenes and tumor-suppressor genes. The
chromosomal aberrations get worse with each cell division eventually producing a cancer cell.

D. **ALL-ANEUPLOIDY THEORY (Figure 11-4).**
The all-aneuploidy theory suggests that cancer
is the result of **aneuploidy** (i.e., abnormal
number of chromosomes) that occurs during
cell division. Although a great majority of aneuploid cells undergo apoptosis, the few sur-
viving cells will produce progeny that are also

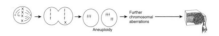

● Figure 11-4 All-Aneuploidy Theory.

aneuploid. The chromosomal aberrations get worse with each cell division eventually
producing a cancer cell.

E. **THE FORMATION OF CANCER STEM CELLS.** All adult tissues contain **adult stem
cells** that are predominately dormant until they are activated when adult tissues require replenishment due to wear and tear or injury. However, the repair capacity of
adult stem cells is limited in comparison with **embryonic stem cells.** Consequently,
when the repair capacity of adult stem cells is exhausted, they may undergo transformation leading to oncogenesis.

Ⅱ The Progression of Cancer

A. **HIGH LEVELS OF GENOMIC INSTABILITY.** Genomic instability is broadly classified
into microsatellite instability (MIN) and chromosome instability (CIN).
1. **Microsatellite instability.** MIN refers to a condition whereby microsatellite DNA
is abnormally lengthened or shortened due to defects in various DNA repair
processes.
2. **Chromosome instability.** CIN refers to condition whereby chromosomal DNA
continuously forms novel chromosome mutations at a rate higher than normal cells.
CIN is typically associated with the accumulation of mutations in proto-oncogenes
and tumor–suppressor genes. The mechanisms of CIN involve chromosome breakage, concurrent breaks in two chromosomes giving rise to translocations, and loss
of chromosomes.

B. **DNA REPAIR.** There are three types of DNA repair that may affect the mutation
phenotype.
1. **Nucleotide excision repair**
2. **Base excision repair**
3. **Mismatch repair (MMR)**

C. **ACCUMULATION OF MUTATIONAL EVENTS.** Currently, it is believed that multiple
mutation events are required to transform normal cells to cancer cells. The current con-
sensus is that oncogenesis imparts six "superpowers" to a cancer cell as indicated below.
1. A cancer cell can grow in the absence of normal growth-promoting signals (e.g.,
EGF [epidermal growth factor]) binding to the EGFR (EGF receptor).

2. A cancer cell can grow in the presence of normal growth-inhibiting signals issued by neighboring cells.

3. A cancer cell CANNOT activate apoptosis (i.e., programmed cell death; "cell suicide") in response to DNA damage.

4. A cancer cell can stimulate blood vessel formation (i.e., angiogenesis).

5. A cancer cell can acquire telomerase activity and become immortalized (i.e., no mitotic limit).

6. A cancer cell can alter its cell membrane receptors to metastasize into other areas of the body.

D. CIN and defects in the MMR pathway are responsible for a variety of hereditary cancer predisposition syndromes including **hereditary nonpolyposis colorectal carcinoma, Bloom syndrome, ataxia-telangiectasia, and Fanconi anemia.**

E. **Epigenetic factors** have emerged to be equally damaging to the cell cycle control. In this regard, **hypermethylation** of promoter regions for tumor-suppressor genes and MMR genes cause **gene silencing** that contributes to oncogenesis.

III. Signal Transduction Pathways. The consequence of an imbalance between the mechanisms of cell cycle control and mutation rates within genes is either the **upregulation of pro-oncogenic signal transduction pathways** or the **downregulation of anti-oncogenic signal transduction pathways.** Some of the common signal transduction pathways that are involved in oncogenesis or oncoprogression are indicated below.

A. MITOGEN-ACTIVATED PROTEIN KINASE PATHWAY (Figure 11-5)

B. TRANSFORMING GROWTH FACTOR PATHWAY (Figure 11-6)

C. PHOSPHATIDYLINOSITOL 3-KINASE/PTEN/AKT PATHWAY (Figure 11-7)

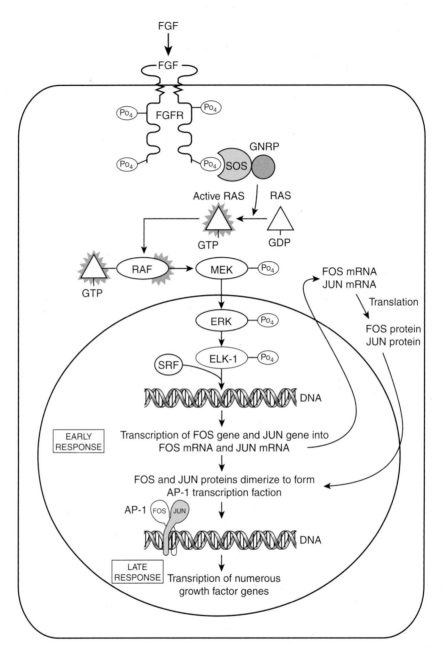

● **Figure 11-5 Mitogen-activated protein kinase (MAPK) pathway.**
- When FGF (fibroblast growth factor) binds to FGFR (fibroblast growth factor receptor), autophosphorylation (PO_4) of FGFR occurs.
- This is recognized by SOS adaptor protein which activates GNRP (guanine nucleotide releasing factor).
- GNRP (guanine nucleotide releasing factor) activates the G-protein RAS by transforming the bound GDP to GTP (RAS-GDP → active RAS-GTP).
- Active RAS-GTP attracts RAF kinase to the inner leaflet of the cell membrane and binds RAF kinase causing a three-dimensional configurational change which activates RAF kinase.
- Active RAF kinase phosphorylates MEK kinase.
- Phosphorylated MEK kinase phosphorylates ERK kinase.
- Phosphorylated ERK kinase enters the nucleus and phosphorylates the transcription factor ELK-1.
- Phosphorylated ELK-1 complexes with SRF (serum response factor) leading to the transcription of **immediate early genes** (called the early response), such as the *FOS* gene and *JUN* gene.
- *FOS* and *JUN* mRNAs exit the nucleus and undergo translation to the FOS and JUN proteins.
- FOS and JUN proteins enter the nucleus and dimerize to form the AP-1 transcription factor.
- The AP-1 transcription factor leads to the transcription of **late response genes** (called the late response). The late response genes include numerous growth factor genes.

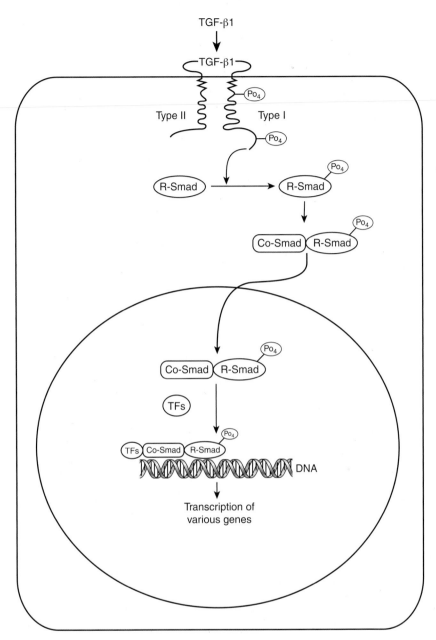

● **Figure 11-6 SMAD (Sma protein and Mad protein) pathway.**
- TGFβ1 is a cytokine which acts as a tumor suppressor in the early stages of oncogenesis through the SMAD pathway.
- When TGF-β binds to the Type II TGF-β receptor, the Type II TGF-β receptor binds the Type I TGF-β receptor and phosphorylates it.
- The phosphorylated Type I and Type II TGF-β receptor complex phosphorylates the R-Smad protein (receptor-regulated Smad protein).
- The phosphorylated R-Smad protein binds to Co-Smad protein (common partner Smad).
- The heterodimeric Smad complex enters the nucleus.
- The Smad complex works with other transcription factors.
- This leads to the transcription of various genes some of which trigger apoptosis.

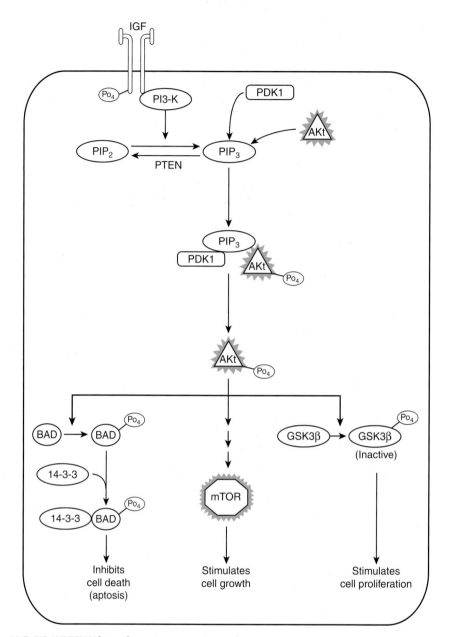

● **Figure 11-7 PI3-K/PTEN/Akt pathway.**

- When IGF (insulin-like growth factor) binds to IGFR (insulin-like growth factor receptor), autophosphorylation (PO_4) of IGFR occurs.
- PI3-K (phosphatidylinositol 3-kinase) binds to IGFR-PO_4 and catalyzes the conversion of PIP_2 (phosphatidylinositol 3, 4 biphosphate) to PIP_3 (phosphatidylinositol 3, 4, 5 triphosphate).
- PTEN (phosphatase and tensin homolog) catalyzes the conversion of PIP_3 to PIP_2. This dephosphorylation is important because it inhibits the PI3-K/PTEN/Akt pathway.
- PIP_3 recruits and serves as a docking site for Akt kinase (transforming retrovirus isolated from the Ak mouse strain) and PDK1 (phosphoinositide-dependent protein kinase).
- Akt is phosphorylated by PDK1 and thereby activated.
- Activated Akt dissociates from the cell membrane and can affect a myriad of substrates via its kinase activity. Three possible pathways are shown.
  - Activated Akt phosphorylates BAD (bcl-xl/bcl-2-antagonist which stimulates cell death). Protein 14-3-3 binds to BAD-PO_4 which sequesters BAD. Sequestered BAD **inhibits cell death (or apoptosis).**
  - Activated Akt activates mTOR kinase (mammalian target of rapamycin) through a series of steps (not shown). Activated mTOR **stimulates cell growth** by increasing protein synthesis.
  - Activated Akt phosphorylates GSK3β (glycogen synthase kinase 3). GSK3β-PO_4 is inactive. Inactive GSK3β-PO_4 **stimulates cell proliferation** by increasing β-catenin levels (the penultimate downstream mediator of the WNT signal pathway) and by increasing protein synthesis.

Chapter 12

Cell Biology of the Immune System

❶ Neutrophils (Polys, Segs, or PMNs) (Figure 12-1)

A. Neutrophils are the most abundant leukocyte in the peripheral circulation (50%–70%).

B. Neutrophils have a multilobed nucleus.

C. Neutrophils have larger primary (azurophilic) granules, which are **endolysosomes** that contain **acid hydrolases** and **myeloperoxidase** (produces hypochlorite ions).

D. Neutrophils have smaller secondary granules that contain **lysozyme, lactoferrin** (participates in free radical generation), **alkaline phosphatase, elastase,** and other **bacteriostatic and bacteriocidal substances.** These substances are mainly released into the extracellular environment.

E. Neutrophils have **respiratory burst oxidase** (a membrane-associated enzyme), which produces hydrogen peroxide (H_2O_2) and superoxide, which kill bacteria.

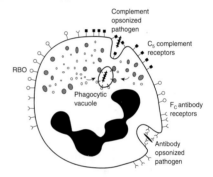

● **Figure 12-1 Neutrophil.** RBO = respiratory burst oxidase.

F. Neutrophils are the first to arrive at an area of tissue damage (within 30 minutes; **acute inflammation**), being attracted to the site by complement C5a and LTB_4. *The Complement System consists of 20 plasma proteins synthesized by the liver that enhance the effect of antibody binding to pathogens (called **opsonization**) so that neutrophils and macrophages may phagocytosed them more easily.*

G. Neutrophils are highly adapted for **anaerobic glycolysis** with large amounts of **glycogen** to function in a devascularized area.

H. Neutrophils play an important role in **PHAGOCYTOSIS of bacteria and dead cells** by using F_C antibody receptors, C5 complement receptors, and bacterial lipopolysaccharides to bind to the foreign material. Neutrophils must bind to the foreign material to begin phagocytosis forming a **phagocytic vacuole.** The primary granules (mainly) and secondary granules bind to the phagocytic vacuole and release their contents to kill the foreign microorganism.

I. Neutrophils impart **natural (or innate) immunity** along with macrophages and natural killer (NK) cells.

J. Neutrophils have a lifespan of **6–10 hours; 2–3 days in tissues.**

II Eosinophils (Figure 12-2)

A. Eosinophils comprise 0%–4% of the leukocytes in the peripheral circulation.

B. Eosinophils have a bilobed nucleus.

C. Eosinophils have highly eosinophilic granules that contain **major basic protein** (MBP; binds to and disrupts membrane of parasites), **eosinophil cationic protein** (works with MBP), **histaminase**, and **peroxidase**.

D. Eosinophils have **immunoglobulin E (IgE)** antibody receptors.

E. Eosinophils play a role in **parasitic infection** (e.g., schistosomiasis, ascariasis, trichinosis).

F. Eosinophils play a role in **reducing the severity of allergic reactions** by secreting histaminase and PGE_1 and PGE_2, which degrades histamine (secreted by mast cells) and which inhibits mast cell secretion, respectively. A large number of eosinophils are found in asthma patients.

G. Eosinophils have a lifespan of **1–10 hours; up to 10 days in tissues**.

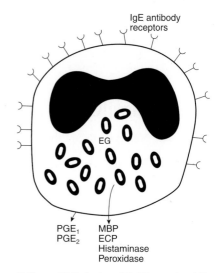

● **Figure 12-2 Eosinophil.** EG = eosinophilic granules; MBP = major basic protein; ECP = eosinophilic cationic protein.

III Basophils (Figure 12-3)

A. Basophils comprise 0%–2% of the leukocytes in the peripheral circulation (i.e., the least abundant leukocyte).

B. Basophils have highly basophilic granules that contain **heparin, histamine, 5-hydroxytryptamine**, and **sulfated proteoglycans**.

C. Basophils have IgE antibody receptors.

D. Basophils play a role in **Type I hypersensitivity anaphylactic reactions** causing **allergic rhinitis (hay fever), some forms of asthma, urticaria**, and **anaphylaxis**.

E. Basophils have a lifespan of **1–10 hours; variable in tissues**.

IV Mast Cells (Figure 12-4)

A. Mast cells arise from stem cells in the bone marrow.

B. Mast cells play a role in **Type I hypersensitivity anaphylactic reactions, inflammation**, and **allergic reactions**.

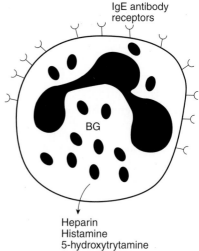

● **Figure 12-3 Basophil.** BG = basophilic granules.

C. Mast cells have **IgE antibody receptors** on their cell membranes that **bind IgE** produced by plasma cells upon **first exposure** to an allergen (e.g., plant pollen, snake venom, foreign serum), which sensitizes the mast cells.

D. Mast cells secrete the following substances upon **second exposure** to the same allergen, causing the classic **wheal-and-flare reaction** in the skin:

  1. Heparin, which is an anticoagulant and cofactor for lipoprotein lipase.

  2. Histamine (produced by decarboxylation of histidine), which increases vascular permeability, causes vasodilation, causes smooth muscle contraction of bronchi, and stimulates HCl secretion from parietal cells in the stomach.

  3. Leukotriene C_4 and D_4 (are eicosanoids and components of slow-reacting substance of anaphylaxis), which increase vascular permeability, cause vasodilation, and cause smooth muscle contraction of bronchi.

  4. Eosinophil chemotactic factor, which attracts eosinophils to the inflammation site.

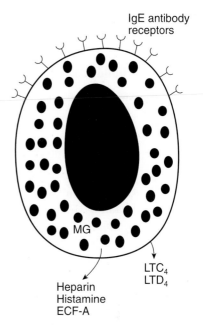

● **Figure 12-4 Mast cell.** MG = mast cell granules; ECF-A = eosinophilic chemotactic factor; LTC_4 = leukotriene C_4; LTD_4 = leukotriene D_4.

Monocytes (Figure 12-5)

A. Monocytes comprise 2%–9% of the leukocytes in the peripheral circulation.

B. Monocytes migrate into peripheral tissues where they differentiate into tissue-specific macrophages whose function is PHAGOCYTOSIS and ANTIGEN PRESENTATION.

C. Monocytes are members of the monocyte-macrophage system, which includes Kupffer cells in liver, alveolar macrophages, macrophages (histiocytes) in connective tissue, microglia in brain, Langerhans cells in skin, osteoclasts in bone, and dendritic antigen-presenting cells (APCs).

D. Monocytes have granules that are endolysosomes that contain acid hydrolases, aryl sulfatase, acid phosphatase, and peroxidase.

E. Monocytes respond to dead cells, microorganisms, and inflammation by leaving the peripheral circulation to enter tissues and are then called macrophages.

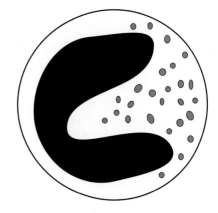

● **Figure 12-5 Monocyte.**

F. Monocytes have a lifespan of 1–3 days; circulate in blood for 12–100 hours, and then enter connective tissue.

VI Macrophages (Histiocytes; Antigen-Presenting Cells) (Figure 12-6)

A. Macrophages arise from **monocytes** within the circulating blood and bone marrow.

B. Macrophages are activated by **lipopolysaccharides** (a surface component of gram-negative bacteria) and **interferon-γ (IFN-γ)**.

C. Macrophages secrete **interleukin-1** (IL-1; stimulates mitosis of T lymphocytes), **interleukin-6** (IL-6; stimulates differentiation of B lymphocytes into plasma cells), **pyrogens** (mediate fever), **tumor necrosis factor-α (TNF-α)**, and **granulocyte-macrophage colony-stimulating factor (GM-CSF)**.

D. Macrophages have granules that are endolysosomes that contain **acid hydrolases, aryl sulfatase, acid phosphatase**, and **peroxidase**.

E. Macrophages impart natural (innate) immunity along with neutrophils and NK cells.

● **Figure 12-6 Macrophage.** LPS = lipopolysaccharide; TNF-α = tumor necrosis factor-α; GM-CSF = granulocyte-macrophage colony-stimulating factor.

F. MACROPHAGES HAVE A PHAGOCYTIC FUNCTION

1. **F_C antibody receptors** on the macrophage cell membrane bind antibody-coated foreign material and subsequently phagocytose the material for lysosomal digestion.
2. **C3 (a component of complement) receptors** on the macrophage cell membrane bind bacteria and subsequently phagocytose the bacteria (called opsonization) for lysosomal digestion.
3. Certain phagocytosed material (e.g., bacilli of tuberculosis and leprosy, Trypanosoma cruzi, Toxoplasma, Leishmania, asbestos) cannot undergo lysosomal digestion, so macrophages will fuse to form **foreign body giant cells**.
4. In sites of chronic inflammation, macrophages may assemble into epithelial-like sheets called **epithelioid cells of granulomas**.

G. MACROPHAGES HAVE AN ANTIGEN-PRESENTING FUNCTION

1. **Exogenous antigens** circulating in the bloodstream are phagocytosed by macrophages and undergo degradation in phagolysosomes.
2. Antigen proteins are degraded into **antigen peptide fragments**, which are presented on the macrophage cell surface in conjunction with **class II major histocompatibility complex (MHC)**.
3. **$CD4^+$ helper T cells** with antigen-specific T-cell receptor (TCR) on its cell surface recognize the antigen peptide fragment.

VII # Natural Killer CD16⁺ Cell (Figure 12-7)

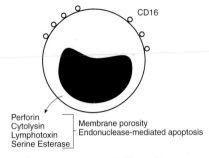

A. The NK cell **is** a member of the **null cell population** (i.e., lymphocytes that do not express the TCR or cell membrane immunoglobulins that distinguish lymphocytes as either T cells or B cells, respectively).

B. NK cells are CD16$^+$ and capable of cytotoxicity without prior antigen sensitization.

C. NK cells attack damaged cells, virus-infected cells, and tumor cells by release of **perforins, cytolysins, lymphotoxins,** and **serine esterases** which cause membrane porosity and endonuclease-mediated apoptosis of the damaged cell, virus-infected cell, or tumor cell.

● **Figure 12-7 Natural killer cell.**

D. They impart natural (innate) immunity along with neutrophils and macrophages.

 VIII # B Lymphocyte (Figure 12-8). In the early fetal development, B-cell lymphopoiesis (B-cell formation) occurs in the **fetal liver.** In later fetal development and throughout the rest of adult life, B-cell lymphopoiesis occurs in the bone marrow. In humans, the **bone marrow is considered the primary site of B-cell lymphopoiesis.**

A. HEMOPOIETIC STEM CELLS originating in the bone marrow differentiate into **lymphoid progenitor cells** which later form **B stem cells.**

B. B stem cells form **Pro-B cells** which begin heavy chain gene rearrangement.

C. PRE-B CELLS continue heavy chain gene rearrangement.

D. IMMATURE B CELLS (IgM$^+$) begin light chain gene rearrangement and express **antigen-specific IgM** (i.e., will recognize only one antigen) on its cell surface.

E. MATURE (OR VIRGIN) B CELLS (IgM$^+$ IgD$^+$) express **antigen-specific IgM and IgD** on their cell surface. Mature B cells migrate to the **outer cortex of lymph nodes, lymphatic follicles in the spleen,** and **gut-associated lymphoid tissue (GALT)** to await antigen exposure.

F. EARLY IMMUNE RESPONSE
1. Early in the immune response, mature B cells bind antigen using IgM and IgD.
2. As a consequence of antigen binding, two transmembrane proteins (**CD79a and CD79b**) that function as signal transducers cause proliferation and differentiation of B cells into **plasma cells that secrete either IgM or IgD.**

G. LATER IMMUNE RESPONSE
1. Later in the immune response, **APCs (macrophages)** phagocytose the antigen where it undergoes lysosomal degradation in **endolysosomes** to form antigen peptide fragments.
2. The **antigen peptide fragments** become associated with the class **II MHC** and are transported and exposed on the cell surface of the APC.
3. The antigen peptide fragment + class II MHC on the surface of the APC is recognized by **CD4$^+$ helper T cells** which secrete **IL-2** (stimulates proliferation of B and T cells), **IL-4 and IL-5** (activate antibody production by causing B-cell differentiation into plasma cells and promote isotype switching and hypermutation), **TNF-α** (activates macrophages), and **IFN-γ** (activates macrophages and NK cells).

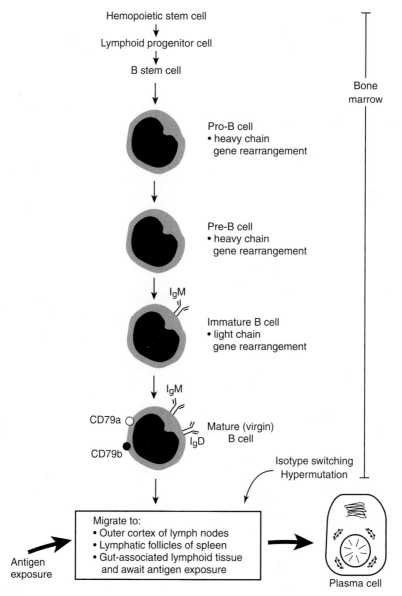

Hemopoietic stem cell

Lymphoid progenitor cell

B stem cell

Pro-B cell
• heavy chain
  gene rearrangement

Pre-B cell
• heavy chain
  gene rearrangement

IgM

Immature B cell
• light chain
  gene rearrangement

IgM

CD79a

Mature (virgin)
IgD   B cell

CD79b

Bone
marrow

Isotype switching
Hypermutation

Migrate to:
• Outer cortex of lymph nodes
• Lymphatic follicles of spleen
• Gut-associated lymphoid tissue
  and await antigen exposure

Antigen
exposure

Plasma cell

● Figure 12-8 B-cell lymphopoiesis.

4. Under the influence of IL-4 and IL-5, mature B cells undergo **isotype switching** and **hypermutation**.

a. **Isotype switching** is a gene rearrangement process whereby the μ (mu; M) and δ (delta; D) **constant segments** of the heavy chain (C_H) are spliced out and replaced with γ (gamma; G), ε (epsilon; E), or α (alpha; A) C_H segments. This allows mature B cells to differentiate into **plasma cells that secrete IgG, IgE, or IgA**.

b. **Hypermutation** is a mutation process whereby a high rate of mutations occurs in the **variable segments** of the heavy chain (V_H) and light chain (V_κ or V_λ). This allows mature B cells to differentiate into plasma cells that secrete IgG, IgE, or IgA that will bind antigen with greater and greater affinity.

IX **T Lymphocyte (Figure 12-9).** In the early fetal development, T-cell lymphopoiesis (T-cell formation) occurs in the **thymic cortex.**

A. HEMOPOIETIC STEM CELLS differentiate into **lymphoid progenitor cells** which form **T stem cells** within the bone marrow.

B. Under the influence of **thymotoxin,** T stem cells leave the bone marrow and enter the thymic cortex where they differentiate into **pre-T cells.** Pre-T cells begin TCR gene rearrangement and express TCR.

C. IMMATURE T CELLS express TCR, CD4, and CD8 and undergo positive or negative selection under the influence of thymosin, serum thymic factor, and thymopoietin.

    1. Positive selection is a process whereby $CD4^+$ $CD8^+$ T cells bind with a certain affinity to MHC proteins expressed on thymic epitheliocytes such that the $CD4^+$ $CD8^+$ T cells become "**educated**"; all other $CD4^+$ $CD8^+$ T cells undergo apoptosis. This means that a mature T cell will respond to antigen only when presented by an MHC protein that it encountered at this stage in its development. This is known as **MHC restriction of T-cell responses.**

    2. Negative selection is a process whereby $CD4^+$ $CD8^+$ T cells interact with thymic dendritic cells at the cortico-medullary junction of the thymus such that $CD4^+$ $CD8^+$ T cells that recognize "self" antigens undergo apoptosis (or are somehow inactivated) leaving only $CD4^+$ $CD8^+$ T cells that recognize only foreign antigens.

D. MATURE T CELLS downregulate CD4 or CD8 to form $CD4^+$ helper T cells, $CD4^+$ or $CD8^+$ suppressor T cells, or $CD8^+$ cytotoxic T cells.

E. Mature T cells migrate to the **paracortex (thymic-dependent zone) of all lymph nodes, periarterial lymphatic sheath in the spleen, and GALT** to await antigen exposure.

F. EXOGENOUS ANTIGENS (circulating in the bloodstream).

    1. Exogenous antigens are internalized by **APCs** and then undergo lysosomal degradation in **endolysosomes** to form antigen peptide fragments.

    2. The antigen peptide fragments become associated with **Class II MHC,** transported, and exposed on the cell surface of the APC.

    3. The antigen peptide fragment + MHC Class II on the surface of the APC is recognized by $CD4^+$ **helper T cells** which secrete **IL-2** (stimulates proliferation of B and T cells), **IL-4** and **IL-5** (activate antibody production by causing B-cell differentiation into plasma cells and promote isotype switching and hypermutation), **TNF-α** (activates macrophages), and **IFN-γ** (activate macrophages and NK cells).

G. ENDOGENOUS ANTIGENS (virus or bacteria within a cell).

    1. Endogenous antigens undergo proteosomal degradation in **proteosomes** within the infected cell to form antigen peptide fragments.

    2. The antigen peptide fragments become associated with **Class I MHC,** transported, and exposed on the cell surface of the infected cell.

    3. The antigen peptide fragment + Class I MHC on the surface of the infected cell is recognized by $CD8^+$ **cytotoxic T cells,** which secrete **perforins, cytolysins, lymphotoxins,** and **serine esterases** which cause membrane porosity and endonuclease-mediated apoptosis of the infected cell.

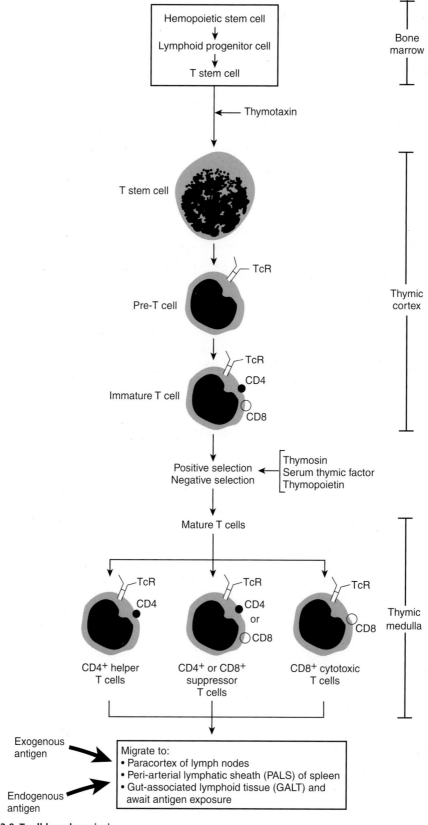

● **Figure 12-9 T-cell lymphopoiesis.**

Immune Response to Exogenous Protein Antigens (Figure 12-10). The

immune response to exogenous protein antigens involves three cells: the mature B cell, an APC, and a CD4$^+$ helper T cell resulting in an early response and a late response to an antigen (X).

A. EARLY RESPONSE

1. Early in the immune response, mature B cells bind antigen using IgM and IgD.
2. As a consequence of antigen binding, two transmembrane proteins (**CD79a and CD79b**) that function as signal transducers cause proliferation and differentiation of B cells into **plasma cells that secrete either IgM or IgD**.

B. LATE RESPONSE

1. Later in the immune response, **APCs (macrophages)** phagocytose the antigen (X) where it undergoes lysosomal degradation in **endolysosomes** to form antigen peptide fragments.
2. The **antigen peptide fragments** become associated with the **class II MHC** and are transported and exposed on the cell surface of the APC.

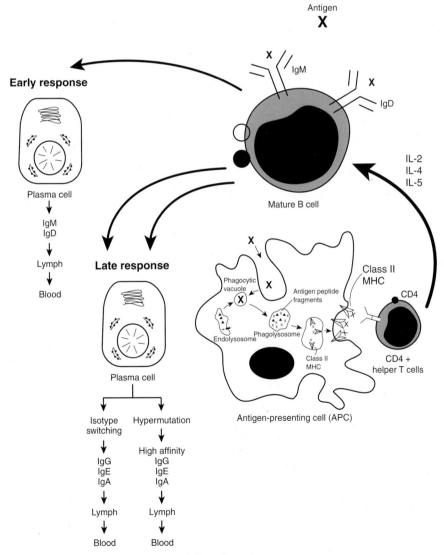

● **Figure 12-10 Immune response to exogenous protein antigen.**

3. The antigen peptide fragment + class II MHC on the surface of the APC is recognized by **CD4$^+$ helper T cells** which secrete.
    a. **IL-2** which stimulates proliferation of B and T cells
    b. **IL-4 and IL-5** which activate antibody production by causing B-cell differentiation into plasma cells and promote isotype switching and hypermutation
    c. **TNF-α** which activates macrophages
    d. **IFN-γ** which activates macrophages and NK cells
4. Under the influence of IL-4 and IL-5, mature B cells undergo **isotype switching** and **hypermutation**.
    a. **Isotype switching** is a gene rearrangement process whereby the μ (mu; M) and δ (delta; D) **constant segments** of the heavy chain (C_H) are spliced out and replaced with γ (gamma; G), ε (epsilon; E), or α (alpha; A) C_H segments. This allows mature B cells to differentiate into **plasma cells that secrete IgG, IgE, or IgA.**
    b. **Hypermutation** is a mutation process whereby a high rate of mutations occurs in the **variable segments** of the heavy chain (V_H) and light chain ($V_κ$ or $V_λ$). This allows mature B cells to differentiate into plasma cells that secrete IgG, IgE, or IgA that will bind antigen with greater and greater affinity.

XI Immune Response to Endogenous Antigens (Intracellular Virus or Bacteria; Figure 12-11)

A. This figure shows the immune response to the hepatitis B virus infecting a hepatocyte of the liver.

B. The viral DNA enters the hepatocyte nucleus and uses the hepatocyte machinery to produce viral mRNA and viral proteins.

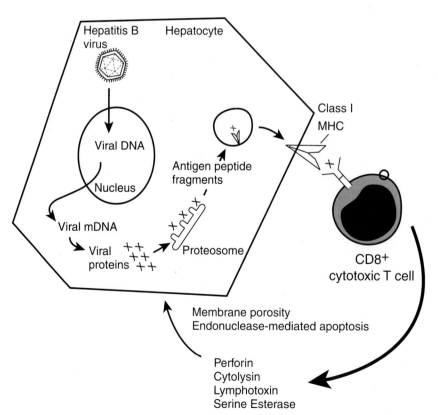

● **Figure 12-11 Immune response to endogenous antigen.**

C. The viral proteins undergo proteosomal degradation in **proteosomes** within the hepatocyte to form antigen peptide fragments.

D. The antigen peptide fragments become associated with the **Class I MHC** and are transported and exposed on the cell surface of the infected cell.

E. The antigen peptide fragment + class I MHC on the surface of the infected cell is recognized by **CD8$^+$ cytotoxic T cells** which secrete **perforin, cytolysins, lymphotoxins,** and **serine esterases** which cause membrane porosity and endonuclease-mediated apoptosis of the infected hepatocyte.

XII Cytokines (Table 12-1)

A. PROPERTIES

1. Cytokines are small, soluble, secreted proteins that enable immune cells to communicate with each other and therefore play an integral role in the initiation, perpetuation, and downregulation of the immune response.

2. Cytokine activity demonstrates **redundancy** and **pleiotropy**. Cytokine redundancy means that many different cytokines may elicit the same activity. Cytokine pleiotropy means that a single cytokine can cause multiple activities.

3. Cytokines act in an **autocrine manner** (i.e., they act on cells that secrete them) or a **paracrine manner** (i.e., they act on nearby cells).

4. Cytokines are often produced in a **cascade** (i.e., one cytokine stimulates its target cell to produce additional cytokines).

5. Cytokines may act **synergistically** (i.e., two or more cytokines acting with one another) or **antagonistically** (i.e., two or more cytokines acting against one another).

B. CYTOKINE RECEPTORS. Cytokines elicit their activity by binding to **high-affinity cell surface receptors** on target cells thereby initiating an intracellular **signal transduction pathway**. Cytokine receptors have been grouped into several families which include the following:

1. Hematopoietin family of receptors. This family of receptors is characterized by four conserved cysteine residues and a conserved Trp-Ser-X-Trp-Ser sequence in the extracellular domain. These receptors generally have two subunits, an **α-subunit** for cytokine binding and a **β-subunit** for signal transduction. Cytokine binding promotes **dimerization** of the α-subunit and β-subunit. This family of receptors binds IL-2, IL-3, IL-4, IL-5, IL-6, IL-7, erythropoietin, and GM-CSF.

2. IFN family of receptors. This family of receptors is characterized by four conserved cysteine residues but does not have a conserved Trp-Ser-X-Trp-Ser sequence in the extracellular domain. This family of receptors binds IFN-α, IFN-β, IFN-γ.

3. TNF family of receptors. This family of receptors is characterized by four extracellular domains. This family of receptor binds TNF-α, TNF-β, membrane-bound CD40, and Fas (which signals a cell to undergo apoptosis).

4. Seven-pass transmembrane helix family of receptors. This family of receptors is characterized by seven transmembrane domains and the interaction with G-proteins. This family of receptors binds IL-8, MIP-1 (macrophage inflammatory protein), and MCP-1 (monocyte chemotactic protein) which are chemokines.

C. CHEMOKINES. Chemokines are chemotactic cytokines that promote chemotaxis (migration) of leukocytes to inflammatory sites. Chemokines are divided into two groups:

1. Chemokines-α or C-X-C chemokines. These chemokines have their first two cysteine residues separated by one amino acid.

2. Chemokines-β or C-C chemokines. These chemokines have two adjacent cysteine residues. This family of receptors is characterized by four conserved cysteine residues and a conserved Trp-Ser-X-Trp-Ser sequence in the extracellular domain.

TABLE 12-1		SELECTED CYTOKINES AND THEIR ACTIVITY	
Cytokine	**Producing Cell**	**Target Cell**	**Activity**
IL-1	Monocytes Macrophages B cells Dendritic cells	T cells B cells Endothelial cells CNS Hepatocytes	Activation of T cells Maturation and proliferation of B cells Increased cell adhesion Fever, sickness behavior Synthesis and release of acute phase proteins
IL-2	T cells	T cells B cells NK cells	Proliferation and differentiation of T cells Proliferation and differentiation of B cells Proliferation and activation of NK cells
IL-4	Th2 cells Mast cells	T cells B cells Macrophages	Proliferation of T cells Isotype switch to IgE by B cells Inhibits IFN-γ activation
IL-6	Th2 cells Macrophages Bone marrow stromal cells Dendritic cells	B cells Plasma cells Hepatocytes Hemopoietic cells	Differentiation into plasma cells Stimulation of antibody secretion Synthesis and release of acute phase proteins Differentiation of hemopoietic cells
IL-8	Macrophages Endothelial cells	All immune cells Endothelial cells	Chemotaxis of all migratory immune cells Activation and chemotaxis of neutrophils Inhibition of histamine release by basophils Inhibition of IgE production by B cells Promotion of angiogenesis
TNF-α	Th1 cells Macrophages Dendritic cells NK cells Mast cells	Virtually all cells in the body	Proinflammatory actions Proliferation of cells Differentiation of cells Cytotoxic for transformed cells

TGF-β	T cells
	Monocytes
		Monocytes
		Macrophages
		B cells
		Various cells of the
		  body
			Chemotaxis of monocytes
			Chemotaxis of macrophages and promotion of
			  IL-1 synthesis
			Promotion of IgA synthesis
			Proliferation of various cells of the body

IFN-γ	Th1 cells
	Cytotoxic T cells
	NK cells
		T cells
		B cells
		Macrophages
			Development of Th1 cells and proliferation of
			  Th2 cells
			Isotype switch to IgG by B cells
			Activation and expression of MHC by
			  macrophages

MCP	Endothelial cells Fibroblasts Smooth muscle cells	Monocytes T cells NK cells Macrophages Basophils Eosinophils	Chemotaxis of monocytes Chemotaxis of T cells Chemotaxis of NK cells Activation of macrophages Promotion of histamine release Activation of eosinophils
MIP	Macrophages	Neutrophils T cells Hematopoietic precursor cells	Chemotaxis of neutrophils Chemotaxis of T cells Inhibition of hematopoiesis
GM-CSF	Th cells	Granulocytes Monocytes Hematopoietic precursor cells	Proliferation and differentiation of granulocytes Proliferation and differentiation of monocytes Proliferation of hematopoietic precursor cells

MCP = monocyte chemotactic protein; MIP = macrophage inflammatory protein; GM-CSF = granulocyte-macrophage colony-stimulating factor; Th = T helper cells; IL = interleukin; IFN = interferon.

Chapter 13

Molecular Biology of the Immune System

I **Clonal Selection Theory.** Clonal selection is the most widely accepted theory that explains the immune system and contains four major points as follows:

A. B cells and T cells of all antigen specificities develop **before exposure to antigen**.

B. Each B cell carries an **immunoglobulin** on its surface for **only a single antigen**; each T cell carries a **T-cell receptor** on its surface for **only a single antigen**.

C. B cells and T cells can be stimulated by antigen to give rise to progeny cells with identical antigen specificity, that is, **clones**.

D. B cells and T cells that are reactive with "self" antigens are eliminated (perhaps through **apoptosis**) or somehow inactivated so that an autoimmune reaction does not occur.

II The B Lymphocyte (B Cell)

A. IMMUNOGLOBULIN (Ig) STRUCTURE (Figure 13-1). An immunoglobulin consists of four protein subunits: **two heavy chains** and **two light chains** that are arranged in a Y-shaped pattern.

1. Heavy chains. The heavy chain gene segments are located on chromosome 14 and include **200 variable segments (V_H), 50 diversity segments (D_H), 6 joining segments (J_H), and 5 constant segments (C_H)**. The 5 C_H segments are named **μ (mu; M), δ (delta; D), γ (gamma; G), ε (epsilon; E), and α (alpha; A)**. The 5 C_H segments define the 5 immunoglobulin classes called IgM, IgD, IgG, IgE, and IgA. The V_H, D_H, J_H, and C_H gene segments undergo gene rearrangement to contribute to immunoglobulin diversity.

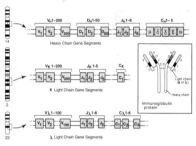

● **Figure 13-1** Immunoglobulin Structure.

2. Light chains

a. **κ (Kappa) chain.** The κ chain gene segments are located on chromosome 2 and include $\approx$200 variable segments (V_κ), 5 joining segments (J_κ), and 1 constant segment (C_κ). The V_κ, J_κ, and C_κ gene segments undergo gene rearrangement to contribute to immunoglobulin diversity.

b. **λ (Lambda) chain.** The λ chain gene segments are located on chromosome 22 and include $\approx$100 variable segments (V_λ), 6 joining segments (J_λ), and 6 constant segments (C_λ). The V_λ, J_λ, and C_λ gene segments undergo gene rearrangement to contribute to immunoglobulin diversity.

3.   The diagram demonstrates immunoglobulin structure. The location of heavy chain and light chain gene segments on chromosomes 14, 2, and 22 are indicated. The heavy and light chain gene segments are organized into various V, D, J, and C gene segments which undergo gene rearrangement, transcription, splicing, and translation to form an immunoglobulin protein. An immunoglobulin protein consists of either two κ light chains or two λ light chains (never a mixture of one κ light chain and one λ light chain). V = variable, D = diversity, J = joining, C = constant.

B.   **IMMUNOGLOBULIN DIVERSITY (Figure 13-2).** For years, the fundamental mystery of the immune system was immunoglobulin diversity: How could B cells (i.e., plasma cells) of the immune system synthesize a million different immunoglobulins, one for each of the million different antigens? If each immunoglobulin was encoded by its own gene, then the human genome would consist almost exclusively of genes dedicated to immunoglobulin synthesis. This is not the case. The answer to this fundamental mystery lies in a number of processes which include the following:

1.   **Gene rearrangement.** The process of gene rearrangement where **V, D, J, and C gene segments of the heavy and light chains are randomly rearranged** in a million combinations that code for a million different immunoglobulins.

2.   **Junctional diversity** whereby DNA deletions occur during gene rearrangement that leads to amino acid changes.

3.   **Insertional diversity** whereby a short sequence of nucleotides in inserted during gene rearrangement that leads to amino acid changes.

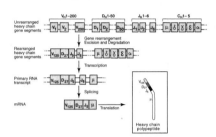

● Figure 13-2 Immunoglobulin Diversity.

4.   **Somatic cell mutations** whereby V gene segments mutate during the life of a B cell.

5.   **Random assortment of heavy and light chains.**

6.   The diagram demonstrates immunoglobulin diversity. The gene rearrangement using heavy chain gene segments as an example is shown. The un-rearranged heavy chain gene segments consisting of 200 V_H segments, 50 D_H segments, 6 J_H segments, and 5 C_H segments undergo gene rearrangement whereby particular segments (V_{125}, $D_{27,}$ and J_5, for example) are brought together while the intervening segments are excised and degraded. The rearranged heavy chain gene segments undergo transcription to form a primary RNA transcript. The primary RNA transcript undergoes splicing to form mRNA (V_{125}, $D_{27,}$ J_5, and μ). The mRNA undergoes translation to form a heavy chain polypeptide with a unique amino acid sequence that corresponds to the V_{125}, $D_{27,}$ J_5, and μ gene segment codons. The gene rearrangement contributes to immunoglobulin diversity. Black segments of the immunoglobulin represent the portion that binds antigen.

C.   **IMMUNOGLOBULIN PROPERTIES (Table 13-1)**

1.   **IgM**

a.   IgM may exist as a **monomer** or **pentamer** structure.

b.   The IgM monomer is synthesized by B cells and retained on the cell membrane of B cells as a B-cell receptor which is specific for a single antigen.

c.   The IgM monomer is designated as $\mu_2 \kappa_2$ or $\mu_2 \lambda_2$.

d.   Later in the immune response, the IgM pentamer is synthesized and secreted by plasma cells. The IgM pentamer is designated as $(\mu_2 \kappa_2)_5$ or $(\mu_2 \lambda_2)_5$ whereby five monomeric IgMs are held together by the **J chain.**

e.   The IgM monomer is a B-cell receptor for antigen.

    f.   The IgM pentamer is the earliest immunoglobulin to appear after antigenic stimulus; activates complement avidly; and does not cross the placenta.

2. IgD. IgD exists as a **monomer.**

    a.   IgD is synthesized by B cells and retained on the cell membrane of B cells as a B-cell receptor which is specific for a single antigen.

    b.   IgD is designated as $\delta_2 \kappa_2$ or $\delta_2 \kappa_2$.

    c.   Later in the immune response, IgD is synthesized and secreted by plasma cells.

    d.   IgD is a B-cell receptor for antigen and an early immunoglobulin to appear after antigenic stimulus; does not activate complement; and does not cross the placenta.

3. IgG

    a.   IgG exists as a **monomer.**

    b.   IgG is synthesized by plasma cells.

    c.   IgG is designated as $\gamma_2 \kappa_2$ or $\gamma_2 \lambda_2$.

    d.   IgG is cleaved into three fragments by **papain** (cleaves above the disulfide bond joining the γ chains) which include **two Fab (fragment; antigen binding) fragments** each containing one reactive site for an antigenic epitope (**monovalent**) and therefore cannot precipitate or agglutinate antigen; **one F_C (fragment; crystallizable) fragment** which activates complement, controls catabolism of IgG, fixes IgG to cells via an F_C receptor on the cell surface, and mediates placental transfer.

    e.   IgG is cleaved into one fragment by **pepsin** which is the **F(ab′)2 fragment** which contains two reactive sites for an antigenic epitope (**bivalent**) and therefore can precipitate or agglutinate antigen; the F_C portion of IgG is extensively digested by pepsin.

    f.   IgG binds to the F_C receptors on neutrophils and macrophages thereby stimulating phagocytosis; activates complement; and crosses the placenta thereby transferring maternal antibodies to the fetus.

4. IgE

    a.   IgE exists as a **monomer**.

    b.   IgE is synthesized by plasma cells.

    c.   IgE is designated as $\varepsilon_2 \kappa_2$ or $\varepsilon_2 \lambda_2$.

    d.   IgE is unstable at 56°C and is called **reagin.**

    e.   IgE binds to IgE antibody receptors on eosinophils, basophils, and mast cells and thereby participates in parasitic infections and Type I hypersensitivity anaphylactic reactions; does not activate complement; and does not cross the placenta.

5. IgA

    a.   IgA exists as a **monomer, dimer,** or **dimer with a secretory piece (called secretory IgA).**

    b.   The **IgA monomer** is synthesized by plasma cells and is found in the serum (little is known about the function of IgA in the serum). The IgA monomer is designated $\alpha_2 \kappa_2$ or $\alpha_2 \lambda_2$.

    c.   The **IgA dimer** is synthesized by plasma cells and is found in the intestinal mucosa. The IgA dimer is designated as $(\alpha_2 \kappa_2)_2$ or $(\alpha_2 \lambda_2)_2$ whereby two monomeric IgAs are held together by the **J chain.**

    d.   The **IgA dimer with secretory piece** is an IgA dimer with a secretory piece (which is a portion of the **poly-Ig receptor complex** found on intestinal epithelial cells) attached to it.

        i.   The IgA dimer synthesized by plasma cells within the lamina propria of the intestinal tract binds to the poly-Ig receptor on the basal surface of the enterocytes to form an **IgA dimer + poly-Ig receptor complex.**

    ii. The IgA dimer + poly-Ig receptor complex is endocytosed and transported across the enterocyte to the apical or luminal surface.

    iii. At the apical surface, the complex is cleaved such that IgA dimer is released into the intestinal lumen joined with the secretory piece of the poly-Ig receptor (called **secretory IgA**). The secretory piece protects IgA dimer from proteolysis.

  e. The IgA dimer is found in high concentrations in external secretions like saliva, mucus, tears, sweat, gastric fluid, and colostrum/milk (provides the neonate with a major source of intestinal protection against pathogens) and works by blocking bacteria, viruses, and toxins from binding to host cells; does not activate complement; and does not cross the placenta.

  f. If all the production of IgA from various sources is taken into account, IgA is the major immunoglobulin in terms of quantity.

D. IMMUNOGLOBULIN FUNCTION. Clearly, the production of immunoglobulins is an important aspect of the immune system. However, the question as to what are the general functions of immunoglobulins that make them so vital needs to be fully understood. The functions of immunoglobulins include the following:

1. **Agglutination.** Agglutination is a process whereby immunoglobulins bind to free antigens to form aggregates that undergo phagocytosis and also reduce the amount of free antigen.

2. **Opsonization.** Opsonization is a process whereby immunoglobulins bind to antigens on the surface of bacteria (for example) which stimulates phagocytosis by neutrophils and macrophages.

3. **Neutralization.** Neutralization is a process whereby immunoglobulins bind to antigen on viruses or bacteria which blocks their adhesion to host cells and inactivates toxins.

4. **Cytotoxicity.** Cytotoxicity is a process whereby immunoglobulins (e.g., IgE) bind to antigen on parasitic worms (e.g., *Schistosoma*) and elicit the eosinophils to release major basic protein, eosinophil cationic protein, histaminase, and peroxidase to kill the worm.

5. **Complement activation.** Complement activation is a process whereby immunoglobulins bind to antigen on the surface of bacteria (for example) which then binds the **proenzyme C′1** of the complement system. This activates the complement cascade resulting in bacterial lysis.

TABLE 13-1	PROPERTIES OF IMMUNOGLOBULINS				
Property	IgM	IgD	IgG	IgE	IgA
H chain	μ	δ	γ	ε	α
L chain	κ or λ	κ or λ	κ or λ	κ or λ	κ or λ
Other chains	J chain	None	None	None	J chain secretory piece (SP)
Structural designation	Monomer: $\mu_2 \kappa_2$ or $\mu_2 \lambda_2$ Pentamer: $(\mu_2 \kappa_2)_5$ or $(\mu_2 \lambda_2)_5$	Monomer: $\delta_2 \kappa_2$ or $\delta_2 \lambda_2$	Monomer: $\gamma_2 \kappa_2$ or $\gamma_2 \lambda_2$	Monomer: $\varepsilon_2 \kappa_2$ or $\varepsilon_2 \lambda_2$	Monomer: $\alpha_2 \kappa_2$ or $\alpha_2 \lambda_2$ Dimer: $(\alpha_2 \kappa_2)_2$ or $(\alpha_2 \lambda_2)_2$ Dimer with SP: $(\alpha_2 \kappa_2)_2$ or $(\alpha_2 \lambda_2)_2$ + SP
Carbohydrate (%)	15	18	4	18	10
Molecular weight (kilodaltons)	Monomer: 180 kDa Pentamer: 950 kDa	Monomer: 184 kDa	Monomer: 150 kDa	Monomer: 188 kDa	Monomer: 160 kDa Dimer: 318 kDa Dimer with SP: 380 kDa
Serum concentration (mg%)	150	3	50–900	0.03	50–300
Serum half-life (days)	5	2.5	8–23	3	6
Binds to F_C receptor	+	−	++	+	−
Activates complement	+++	−	++	−	−
Crosses placenta	No	No	Yes	No	No

The T Lymphocyte (T Cell)

A. T-CELL RECEPTOR (TCR) STRUCTURE (Figure 13-3).
A TCR consists of two protein subunits: 1 α (alpha) chain and 1 β (beta) chain or 1 γ (gamma) chain and 1 δ (delta) chain.

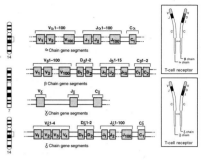

1. **The α chain.** The α chain gene segments are located on chromosome 14 and include 100 variable segments (V_α), 100 joining segments (J_α), and 1 constant segment (C_α), resembling the immunoglobulin light chains. The $V_\alpha, J_\alpha, C_\alpha$ gene segments undergo gene rearrangement to contribute to TCR diversity.

● Figure 13-3 T Cell Receptor Structure.

2. **The β chain.** The β chain gene segments are located on chromosome 7 and include ≈100 variable segments (V_β), 2 diversity segments (D_β), 15 joining segments (J_β), and 2 constant segments (C_β), resembling the immunoglobulin heavy chains. The $V_\beta, D_\beta, J_\beta, C_\beta$ gene segments undergo gene rearrangement to contribute to TCR diversity.

3. **The γ chain.** The γ chain gene segments are located on chromosome 7 and include variable segments (V_γ), joining segments (J_γ), or constant segments (C_γ), resembling the immunoglobulin light chains. The $V_\gamma, J_\gamma, C_\gamma$ gene segments undergo gene rearrangement to contribute to TCR diversity.

4. **The δ chain.** The δ chain gene segments are located on chromosome 14 and include ≈4 variable segments (V_δ), 2 diversity segments (D_δ), 100 joining segments (J_δ), and 1 constant segment (C_δ), resembling the immunoglobulin heavy chains. The $V_\delta, D_\delta, J_\delta, C_\delta$ gene segments undergo gene rearrangement to contribute to TCR diversity.

5. The diagram demonstrates TCR structure. The location of the α chain, β chain, γ chain, and δ chain gene segments on chromosomes 7 and 14 are indicated. The α, β, γ, and δ chain gene segments are organized into various V, D, J, and C gene segments which undergo gene rearrangement, transcription, splicing, and translation to form a TCR. A TCR consists of either a **α chain and β chain (αβ)** or a **γ chain and δ chain (γδ)**. V = variable, D = diversity, J = joining, C = constant.

B. TCR DIVERSITY (Figure 13-4)

1. The fundamental principles of gene rearrangement already explained for immunoglobulins also apply to the diversity found in the TCR.

2. The diagram demonstrates TCR diversity. The gene rearrangement using β chain gene segments as an example is shown. The un-rearranged β chain gene segments consisting of 100 V_β segments, 2 D_β segments, 15 J_β segments, and 2 C_β segments undergo gene rearrangement whereby particular segments (e.g., V_{49}, D_1, J_9, and

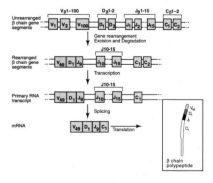

● Figure 13-4 T Cell Receptor Diversity.

C_1) are brought together while intervening gene segments are excised and degraded. The rearranged β chain gene segments undergo transcription to form a primary RNA transcript. The primary RNA transcript undergoes splicing to form mRNA (V_{49}, D_1, J_9, and C_1). The mRNA undergoes translation to form a β chain polypeptide with a unique amino acid sequence that corresponds to the V_{49}, D_1, J_9, and C_1 gene segment codons. Black segments of the TCR represent the portion that binds antigen.

IV Clinical Considerations

A. X-LINKED INFANTILE AGAMMAGLOBULINEMIA (XLA; BRUTON)

1. XLA is caused by a mutation in the *BTK* gene (Bruton tyrosine kinase) located on **chromosome X (Xq22)** which encodes for a **tyrosine kinase** involved in the differentiation of pre-B cells into mature B cells.
2. This disorder is due to the inability of pre-B cells to differentiate into mature B cells due to the **failure of V_H gene segments to undergo gene rearrangement**.
3. Clinical signs include the following: occurs only in male infants, becomes apparent at 5–6 months of age, recurrent **bacterial** otitis media, septicemia, pneumonia, arthritis, meningitis, and dermatitis (most commonly due to *Haemophilus influenza* and *Streptococcus pneumonia*).
4. Laboratory findings include an **absence of all classes of immunoglobulins** within the serum and <1% CD19$^+$ B cells or CD20$^+$ B cells.

B. SEVERE COMBINED IMMUNE DEFICIENCY (SCID).

The SCID syndromes are a heterogeneous group of disorders due to a defect in the development and function of B cells and T cells. In some cases, the defect causes only T-cell dysfunction, but immunoglobulin production may also be compromised because B cells require signals from T cells to produce an effective immunoglobulin response. SCID presents in the early newborn period but can be delayed several months because maternally derived immunoglobulins provide early immune protection.

1. **Adenosine deaminase deficiency (ADA; ADA⁻ SCID)**
   a. ADA is caused by a mutation in the *ADA* gene located on **chromosome 20q12-q13.11** which encodes for **adenosine deaminase** which catalyzes the deamination of adenosine and deoxyadenosine into inosine and deoxyinosine, respectively. Inosine and deoxyinosine are converted to waste products and excreted.
   b. A lack of adenosine deaminase activity results in the **accumulation of adenosine and deoxyadenosine** which are particularly toxic to T cells.
   c. Clinical signs include recurrent severe infections, chronic mucocutaneous candidiasis, infections with common viral pathogens (e.g., respiratory syncytial virus, varicella zoster, herpes simplex, measles, influenza, parainfluenza) are frequently fatal, susceptibility to opportunistic infections (e.g., *Pneumocystis carinii*), attenuated vaccine organisms (e.g., oral polio vaccine virus) may cause fatal infection, chronic diarrhea, and failure to thrive. The only treatment for all forms of SCID is stem cell transplantation.
   d. Laboratory findings include severe T-cell deficiency with low numbers of CD3$^+$ and CD4$^+$ T cells, poor in vitro lymphocyte mitogenic and antigenic responses, and absent mixed lymphocyte reactions.

C. 22Q11.2 DELETION SYNDROME (DS; CONGENITAL THYMIC APLASIA; DIGEORGE SYNDROME)

1. DS is caused by a microdeletion of the **DiGeorge chromosomal critical region** on **chromosome 22q11.2**. Approximately 90% of DS individuals have a de novo deletion.

2. The *TBX1* gene which encodes for **T-box transcription factor TBX10 protein** is most likely one of the genes that is deleted in DS and results in some of the clinical features of DS.

3. DS encompasses the phenotypes previously called **DiGeorge syndrome, velocardiofacial syndrome, conotruncal anomaly face syndrome, Opitz g/BBB syndrome,** and **Cayler cardiofacial syndrome.**

4. These infants have **no T cells** and many infants even fail to mount an immunoglobulin response which requires CD4$^+$ helper T cells.

5. Clinical signs include facial anomalies resembling first arch syndrome (micrognathia, low-set ears) due to abnormal neural crest cell migration, cardiovascular anomalies due to abnormal neural crest cell migration during formation of the aorticopulmonary septum (e.g., Tetralogy of Fallot), velopharyngeal incompetence, cleft palate, immunodeficiency due to thymic hypoplasia, hypocalcemia due to parathyroid hypoplasia, and embryological formation of pharyngeal pouches 3 and 4 fail to differentiate into the thymus and parathyroid glands.

Ⅴ Disorders of Phagocytic Function

A. MYELOPEROXIDASE DEFICIENCY (MPO)

1. MPO (a relatively benign immunodeficiency) is caused by a mutation in the *MPO* gene located on **chromosome 17q23** which encodes for **myeloperoxidase.**

2. Myeloperoxidase catalyzes the conversion of H_2O_2 and chloride ion (Cl^-) into **hypochlorous acid (i.e., bleach).**

3. MPO is most commonly caused by a missense mutation which results in a **normal arginine → tryptophan substitution** at position 569 (R569W).

4. Myeloperoxidase is synthesized by neutrophils and macrophages, packaged in endolysosomes (or azurophilic granules), and released into phagolysosomes or the extracellular space.

5. Clinical signs: most individuals have no increased frequency of infections; if infections due occur, they are usually fungal in nature due to *Candida albicans* or *Candida tropicalis.*

B. CHEDIAK-HIGASHI SYNDROME (CHS)

1. CHS is a rare childhood autosomal recessive genetic disorder caused by a mutation in the *CHS1* gene located on **chromosome 1q42.1–42.2** which encodes for the **CHS protein.**

2. The CHS protein is a **trafficking regulator protein** which is involved in the **formation, fusion, or trafficking of storage/secretory granules** in various cell types (e.g., lysosomes in neutrophils and other leukocytes, dense bodies of platelets, and melanosomes in melanocytes).

3. Clinical signs include recurrent pyogenic infections of the respiratory tract and skin; severe gingivitis; oral mucosa ulceration; partial oculocutaneous albinism; neurological disturbances (e.g., photophobia, nystagmus, peripheral neuropathy, spinocerebellar degeneration, and seizures); **accelerated phase** involves widespread infiltration of lymphocytes and histiocytes into the liver, spleen, and lymph nodes; and few patients live to adulthood.

4. Laboratory findings include neutrophils contain markedly abnormal giant cytoplasmic granules which are formed by the abnormal fusion of endolysosomes with endosomes.

VI Systemic Autoimmune Disorders

A. SYSTEMIC LUPUS ERYTHEMATOUS. See Chapter 6VA.

B. RHEUMATOID ARTHRITIS (RA; Figure 13-5)

1. RA is a chronic, systemic, peripheral polyarthritis of unknown causes that typically leads to deformity and destruction of joints due to erosion of cartilage and bone.

2. RA has an association with **major histocompatibility complex (MHC) Class II genes** located on **chromosome 6**. The association becomes better defined when the **HLA-DRB1 allele** (MHC, Class II, DR beta 1) is evaluated because it appears that this allele is involved in MHC Class II binding antigenic peptides and presented them to CD4$^+$ T cells.

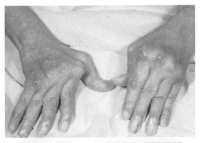

3. All of the associated alleles have in common a **shared epitope** involving amino acids 67–74. Within this shared epitope, a sequence of arginine, alanine, and alanine at position 72–74 (RAA 72–74) appears to account for the majority of increased risk of RA.

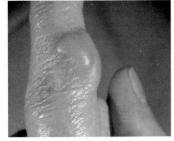

4. Clinical signs include insidious onset; morning stiffness present for at least 1 hour; pain, stiffness and swelling of three

● **Figure 13-5 Rheumatoid Arthritis.**

or more joints; swelling of wrist, metacarpophalangeal or proximal interphalangeal joints; symmetric joint swelling; usually progresses from the peripheral to proximal joints; rheumatoid subcutaneous nodules; may lead to destruction of the joints due to erosion of bone and cartilage; synovial thickening may be detected by a "boggy" feel to the swollen joint.

5. Laboratory findings include anti-CCP antibodies (citrulline-containing proteins).

6. The top photograph shows the hands of a patient with advanced RA. Note the swelling of the metacarpal phalangeal joints and classic ulnar deviation of the fingers. The bottom photograph shows a rheumatoid nodule on a finger.

VII Organ-Specific Autoimmune Disorders

A. BLOOD DISORDERS. **Monoclonal gammopathies** refer to a group of **neoplastic** diseases involving the abnormal proliferation of B cells and plasma cells resulting in excessive production of immunoglobulins or immunoglobulin chains.

1. **Multiple myeloma (MM; Figure 13-6)**

   a. MM is most commonly caused by reciprocal translocation between band q32 on chromosome 14 containing the immunoglobulin heavy chain gene and the following:

      i. Band p16 on chromosome 4 containing the FGF (fibroblast growth factor) receptor 3 gene [t(14;4) (q32;p16)].

ii. Band p25 on chromosome 6 containing the interferon regulatory factor 4 gene [**t(14;6) (q32;p25)**].

iii. Band q13 on chromosome 11 containing the cyclin D1 gene [**t(14;11) (q32;q13)**].

iv. Band q23 on chromosome 16 containing the C-MAF transcription factor [**t(14;16) (q32;q23)**].

b. A common mechanism by which these translocations may lead to MM is unknown.

c. MM is characterized by the malignant proliferation of plasma cells within the bone marrow compartment.

d. The malignant plasma cells produce high levels of a **single monoclonal immunoglobulin** or **free κ chains** or **λ chains** (called **Bence-Jones proteins**) in the serum or urine.

e. MM is the most common type of monoclonal gammopathy.

f. Clinical signs include high susceptibility to bacterial and viral infections since normal immunoglobulin synthesis is suppressed; back and chest bone pain; bone resorption; weakness and fatigue associated with anemia; pallor; radiculopathy; and renal failure.

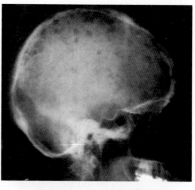

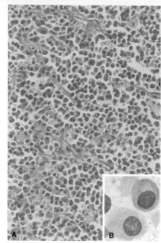

● Figure 13-6 Multiple Myeloma.

g. Laboratory findings include large, waxy, laminated casts in the renal tubules; hypercalcemia; normocytic, normochromic anemia; rouleaux formation; and demonstration of monoclonal Ig (**M proteins**; called the "**M spike**") in the serum or urine by electrophoresis.

h. The top lateral radiograph shows multiple lytic lesions in the calvarium. The bottom light micrograph shows bone marrow from a patient with MM. Note the sheet of atypical plasma cells which vary in size and shape.

B. CENTRAL NERVOUS SYSTEM (CNS) DISORDERS

1. Multiple sclerosis (MS; Figure 13-7)

a. MS is caused by unknown mechanisms.

b. MS is an autoimmune disease of the CNS and is characterized by multifocal areas of demyelination with relative preservation of axons, loss of oligodendrocytes, and astroglial scarring.

c. MS results in paralysis, loss of sensation, and loss of coordination although the exact nature of the defect depends on the specific area of the CNS involved.

d. Clinical signs include the following: affects primarily women of Northern European descent of childbearing age (15–50 years of age); fatigue; sensory loss in limb; visual loss; subacute motor loss; diplopia; polysymptomatic

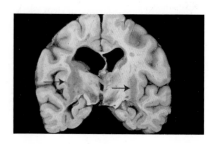

● Figure 13-7 Multiple Sclerosis.

onset; relapses and remissions; optic neuritis; and Lhermitte's sign (sudden, transient, electric-like shocks spreading down the body when the patient flexes the head forward).

e. Laboratory findings include the following: cerebral or spinal plaques which consist of a discrete region of demyelination with relative axonal preservation is seen on MRI; active plaques show perivascular infiltration of T cells and macrophages with occasional plasma cells; gadolinium-DPTA is a paramagnetic contrast agent that crosses a disrupted blood-brain barrier and is used to assess plaque activity (new or newly active plaques accumulate gadolinium); oligoclonal bands which represent limited classes of immunoglobulins (depicted as discrete bands on agarose gels) are found in 85%–95% of MS patients; **antimyelin antibodies** may correlate with MS activity or predict progression from a clinically isolated event to MS although the data are conflicting.

f. The photograph shows a coronal section of the brain with prominent demyelinated plaques (arrows).

2. Myasthenia gravis (MG)

a. MG is caused by unknown mechanisms.

b. MG is an autoimmune disease of the skeletal muscles involving the nicotinic acetylcholine receptor (nAChR) located at the neuromuscular junction.

c. MG is characterized by weakness and fatigability of skeletal muscles.

d. Clinical signs: affects women of 20–30 years of age or men older than 60 years of age; fatigue as the degree of muscle weakness increases with exercise and improvement with rest; muscle weakness often begins with the ocular muscles—however, the facial muscles or limbs muscles may also be initially affected; ptosis; diplopia; "myasthenic snarl" may be observed when facial muscles are affected; nasal speech; difficulty in swallowing; thymic hyperplasia; and thymoma.

e. Laboratory findings: **anti-nAChR antibodies** are present and mediate the physical symptoms; the anti-nAChR antibodies belong to the IgG_1 and IgG_3 subclasses and therefore fix complement; the anti-nAChR antibodies may be directed against any of the five subunits of the nAChR; some patients who are anti-nAChR negative have **anti–muscle-specific receptor tyrosine kinase.**

Chapter 14

Molecular Biology Techniques

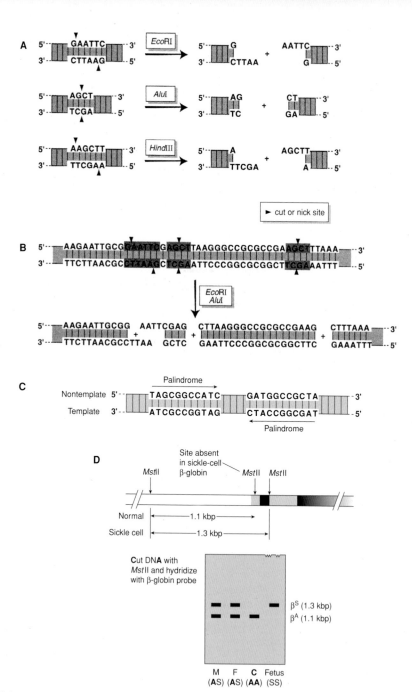

● Figure 14-1

Action of Restriction Enzymes.
Restriction enzymes (REs) are bacterial enzymes that catalyze the **hydrolysis of the phosphodiester bond** in the DNA molecule (i.e., **cut the DNA**) at **specific nucleotide sequences** (4–10 base pairs long). These enzymes are crucial to DNA technology because treatment of a DNA sample with a particular RE will always produce the same pattern of DNA fragments.

Figure 14-1A Action of *Eco*R1, *Alu*1, and *Hind*III. The action (i.e., **hydrolysis of the phosphodiester bond**) of REs *Eco*R1, *Alu*1, and *Hind*III is shown. The **specific nucleotide sequences** that each RE recognizes and its cut site (▲) is indicated. Note that *Eco*R1 and *Hind*III produce DNA fragments with **staggered ends**, whereas *Alu*1 produces DNA fragments with **blunt ends**.

Figure 14-1B Action of *Eco*R1 and *Alu*1 on a long piece of DNA. A long piece of DNA will have many cut sites. If this long piece of DNA is treated with both *Eco*R1 and *Alu*1, the four DNA fragments indicated will always be produced due to the specificity of the REs. You may be asked on the USMLE to deduce the DNA fragments produced in an RE reaction.

Figure 14-1C Palindromes (or inverted repeat sequences). Palindromes are two identical base sequences on different strands on the DNA (i.e., nontemplate strand and template strand) and running in opposite directions (or read the same in the $5' \rightarrow 3'$ direction).

Figure 14-1D Direct detection of the sickle cell anemia mutant β-globin gene:

- Sickle cell anemia is an autosomal recessive genetic disease caused by a mutation in the β-globin gene that results in a change of single amino acid from **glutamic acid** (normal) to **valine** (mutant) in the β-globin protein.
- The base change (A $\rightarrow$ T) destroys the recognition sequence for a number of REs, including *Mst*II.
- *Mst*II cuts the normal β-globin gene into two fragments, **1.1 and 0.2 kb.**
- *Mst*II cuts the mutant β-globin gene into one **1.3 kb** fragment because the A $\rightarrow$ T base change destroys one of the *Mst*II cut sites.
- A Southern blot can be performed on the *Mst*II cut DNA and hybridized with a β-globin probe. The Southern blot shows the prenatal diagnosis of sickle cell anemia using the *Mst*II polymorphism. The mother (M) and father (F) are heterozygote (AS) carriers of sickle cell anemia because they show the l.l and 1.4 kb fragments. Their normal child (C) is homozygous (AA) because he shows only the 1.1 kb fragment. Their fetus is homozygous (SS) and will have sickle cell anemia because the fetus shows only the 1.3 kb fragment.

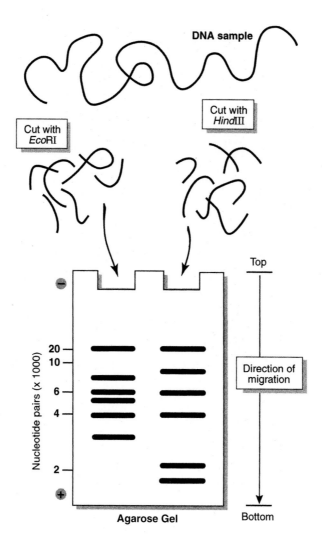

● Figure 14-2

Electrophoresis:

- When separating proteins or small nucleic acids (DNA, RNA, or oligonucleotides), the gel is usually composed of different concentrations of acrylamide and a cross-linker, producing different sized mesh networks of **polyacrylamide**. When separating larger nucleic acids (greater than a few hundred bases), the preferred matrix is purified **agarose**.
- After a DNA sample is cut into fragments by an RE, the DNA fragments can be separated from one another by PAGE based on **size of the DNA fragments.**
- The sizes of the DNA fragments can be compared and a physical map (called a **restriction map**) of the DNA sample can be constructed showing the location of each cut site.
- A DNA sample is cut with either *Eco*R1 or *Hind*III REs.
- The mixture of DNA fragments obtained from the RE treatment is placed at the top of the agarose gel slab and under an electric field, the DNA fragments move through the gel toward the positive electrode because DNA is negatively charged.
- Smaller DNA fragments migrate faster than large DNA fragments and thus the DNA fragments in the mixture become separated by size.
- Note that **smaller DNA fragments** are located at the **bottom of the gel** and **larger DNA fragments** are located at the **top of the gel.**
- To visualize the DNA fragments in the gel, the gel is soaked in a dye that binds to DNA and fluoresces under ultraviolet light.

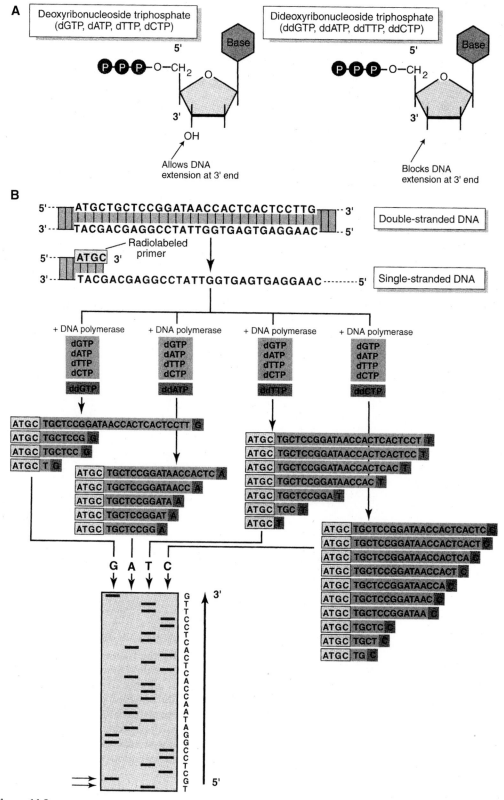

● **Figure 14-3**

The Enzymatic Method of DNA Sequencing.
Although restriction maps provide useful information concerning a DNA sample, the ultimate physical map of DNA is its **nucleotide sequence**. The nucleotide sequence is established by a technique called DNA sequencing. This method employs the use of DNA synthesis with **dideoxyribonucleoside triphosphates** which **lack the 3'-OH group** that is normally found on deoxyribonucleoside triphosphates. If a dideoxyribonucleoside triphosphate becomes incorporated into DNA during synthesis, the addition of the next nucleotide is **blocked** due to the lack of the 3'-OH group. This forms the basis of the enzymatic method of DNA sequencing.

Figure 14-3A The biochemical structure of deoxyribonucleoside triphosphates (dGTP, dATP, dTTP, dCTP) and dideoxyribonucleoside triphosphates (ddGTP, ddATP, ddTTP, ddCTP) is shown. Note the lack of the 3'-OH group on the dideoxyribonucleoside triphosphates.

Figure 14-3B:

- Double-stranded DNA is separated into single strands and one of the strands is used as the template.
- A radiolabeled primer (ATGC) is used to initiate DNA synthesis.
- Four separate reaction mixtures are set up containing DNA polymerase, dGTP, dATP, dTTP, dCTP and ddGTP, ddATP, ddTTP, or ddCTP. These four reactions will produce a number of different length DNA fragments which will terminate in G, A, T, or C depending on what dideoxyribonucleoside triphosphate was present in the reaction mixture.
- The contents of each reaction mixture are separated by gel electrophoresis based on size of the DNA fragments.
- The gel is then exposed to film such that the radiolabeled primer will identify each of the DNA fragments as bands. The bands are arranged as four parallel columns representing DNA fragments of varying lengths that terminate in G, A, T, or C.
- A typical DNA sequencing film is shown and you may be asked on the USMLE to read a sequencing gel.
- Start at the bottom the film and identify the lowest band (i.e., the shortest DNA fragment) and note that the lowest band in found in the T column ($\rightarrow$). Now you know that the first nucleotide in the sequence is T.
- Go the next lowest band on the film and note that it is found under the G column ($\rightarrow$). Now you know that the second nucleotide in the sequence is G.
- Continue this process for all 26 bands.
- Note that when you start at the bottom of the film and go up, you will be constructing the DNA sequence in a **5' $\rightarrow$ 3' direction**.

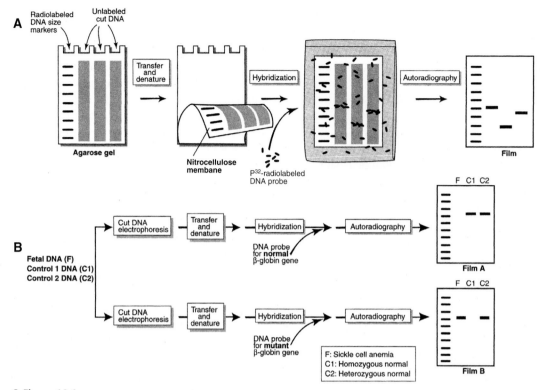

● Figure 14-4

Southern Blotting and Prenatal Testing for Sickle Cell Anemia. Southern blotting

allows for the identification of a **specific DNA sequence** (e.g., gene for the β-globin chain of hemo-globin) by using a **DNA probe** and the **hybridization reaction**. A DNA probe is a single-stranded piece of DNA (10–120 base pairs **oligonucleotide**) that participates in a hybridization reaction. A hybridization reaction is a reaction whereby a single-stranded piece of DNA (like a DNA probe) binds (or hybridizes) with another piece of single-stranded DNA of **complementary nucleotide sequence**. The hybridization reaction exploits a fundamental property of DNA to denature and renature. The two strands of double-helix DNA are held together by **weak hydrogen bonds** that can be broken (denatured) by **high temperature** (90°C) or **alkaline pH** such that single-stranded DNA is formed. Under **low temperature** or **acid pH**, single-stranded DNA will reform double-helix DNA (renature). A Southern blot is used to detect major gene rearrangements and deletions found in a variety of human diseases. A Southern blot can also be used to identify structurally related genes in the same species and homologous genes in other species. Basically, a Southern blot gives information whether a gene is present or absent but does not give information about the expression of the gene.

Figure 14-4A Southern blotting:

- Double-stranded DNA is cut by three different REs and separated by gel electrophoresis in three separate lanes. One lane is reserved for radiolabeled DNA size markers.
- The double-stranded DNA is transferred to a nitrocellulose membrane under alkaline conditions so the DNA is denatured into single strands.
- The nitrocellulose paper is placed in a plastic bag along with the **radiolabeled P^{32} DNA probe** and incubated under conditions that favor hybridization.
- The nitrocellulose paper is exposed to photographic film (autoradiography) so that the radiolabeled probe will show up as bands.

Figure 14-4B Prenatal testing for sickle cell anemia. It is good news when you hear that a gene has been cloned and sequenced because now a DNA probe that hybridizes to the gene can be made and used, for example, in prenatal testing for sickle cell anemia. Sickle cell anemia is a recessive genetic disease caused by a mutation in the β-globin gene that results in a change of single amino acid from **glutamic acid** (normal) to **valine** (mutant) in the β-globin protein. Both the normal gene and mutant gene for β-globin protein have been sequenced so that DNA probes can be made to locate both of these genes in a Southern blot.

- Fetal DNA (F) is obtained from a high-risk fetus and compared with control DNA (C1 & C2). The DNA is separated into two samples. Each sample is cut with REs, subjected to gel electrophoresis, and transferred to nitrocellulose paper under denaturing conditions.
- One sample is hybridized with a DNA probe for the normal β-globin gene and the other sample is hybridized with a DNA probe for the mutant β-globin gene.
- After autoradiography, the films A and B can be analyzed.
- You will likely be asked to interpret a Southern blot on the USMLE for an autosomal recessive, autosomal dominant, or X-linked genetic disease.
- Examine lane F (fetal DNA) in films A and B. Note that lane F has no bands in film A (no normal β-globin gene) but one band in film B (mutant β-globin gene). This means that the fetus is homozygous for the mutant β-globin gene and therefore will have sickle cell anemia.
- Examine lane C1 (control DNA) in films A and B. Note that lane C1 has one band in film A but no bands in film B. This means that this person is homozygous for the normal β-globin gene and therefore will be normal.
- Examine lane C2 (control DNA) in films A and B. Note that lane C2 has one band in film A and one band in film B. This means that this person is heterozygous having one copy of the normal β-globin gene and one copy of the mutant β-globin gene. This person will be normal because sickle cell anemia is genetic recessive disease so that two copies of the mutant β-globin gene are necessary for sickle cell anemia to appear.

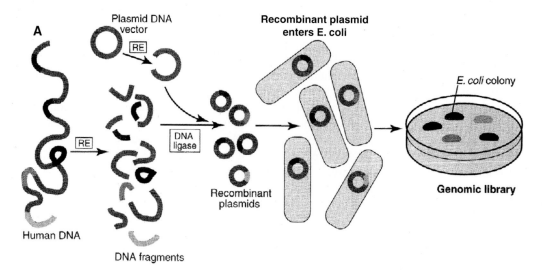

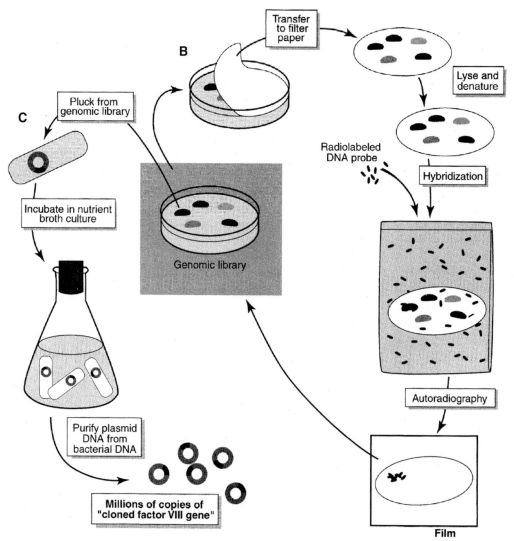

● Figure 14-5

Isolating a Human Gene by DNA Cloning.

The term "cloning" is somewhat confusing because it is used in three ways. First, cloning means making identical copies of a DNA molecule. Second, cloning means isolating a particular gene from the rest of the DNA. Third, human cloning means the creation of a genetically identical copy of a human being, human cell, or human tissue. Although human clones are naturally produced in the form of identical twins, laboratory-produced human cloning is controversial. Artificial therapeutic cloning involves cloning cells from an adult for use in medicine. Artificial reproductive cloning involves making cloned humans and is illegal in many countries.

Although the exact method of cloning differs from gene to gene, we will use the cloning of **human Factor VIII** as an example of a general cloning strategy. The first step in cloning human Factor VIII is the construction of a **genomic library**. The construction of a genomic library employs the use of a **plasmid vector** (or **cloning vector**). A **plasmid vector** is a circular DNA molecule that can infect and replicate inside a bacterium. Plasmid DNA can be combined with human DNA to form a **recombinant plasmid**. A major disadvantage of plasmid vectors is that they accept only small DNA fragments. Consequently, other vectors that accept long DNA fragments have been designed which include **cosmid vectors** based on the bacteriophage λ; **BACs (bacterial artificial chromosomes)** based on the F-factor plasmids; **PACs (P1 artificial chromosomes)** based on the P1 bacteriophage; and **YACs (yeast artificial chromosomes)**.

Figure 14-5A Construction of a genomic library:

- Human DNA is cut with an RE into DNA fragments. A plasmid DNA vector is also cut with the same RE and the two types of DNA are mixed together.
- Human DNA fragments will be inserted into the plasmid DNA and sealed with DNA ligase. This forms a recombinant plasmid, that is, DNA from two different sources has been "recombined."
- **pBR322** is a widely used versatile plasmid that contains two antibiotic resistance genes (ampicillin and tetracycline). The tetracycline gene has a BAMH1 RE site that can be used to insert human DNA fragments into the pBR322 plasmid. This results in bacteria that will be resistant to only ampicillin and will not grow in the presence of tetracycline.
- The recombinant plasmids are mixed with *Escherichia coli* bacteria and plated on Petri plates forming bacterial colonies which constitute a genomic library. Plasmids enter bacteria by **conjugation** (Gram-), **transduction** (most Gram + by using bacteriophages), or **transformation** (using temperature changes or $CaCl_2$).

Figure 14-5B Screening the library:

- Bacteria colonies are transferred to filter paper, lysed, and the DNA is denatured to single strands under alkaline conditions.
- Because a portion of the amino acid sequence of Factor VIII protein was already known, the DNA sequence that codes for these amino acids can be deduced. A DNA probe was made based on this deduced DNA sequence. The radiolabeled DNA probe hybridizes to the DNA strand of complementary nucleotide sequence, that is, the Factor VIII gene.
- The filter paper is exposed to photographic film to identify the radiolabeled DNA.

Figure 14-5C Amplification:

- The corresponding bacterial colony is plucked from the Petri dish and introduced to a nutrient broth culture overnight.
- The recombinant plasmid DNA is separated from the bacterial DNA such that you now have millions of copies of the recombinant plasmid containing the Factor VIII gene.
- Hence, you have cloned the Factor VIII gene.

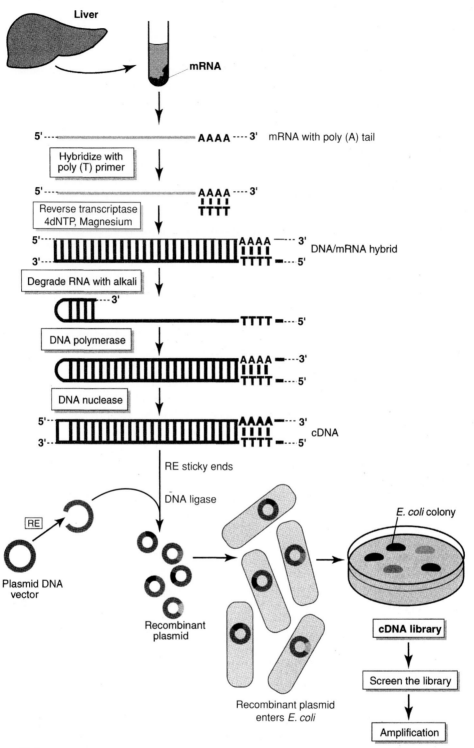

Liver

mRNA

5'----▬▬▬▬▬▬▬▬▬▬▬▬▬▬▬▬AAAA----3' mRNA with poly (A) tail

Hybridize with
poly (T) primer

5'----▬▬▬▬▬▬▬▬▬▬▬▬▬▬▬AAAA----3'
TTTT

Reverse transcriptase
4dNTP, Magnesium

5'----AAAA----3' DNA/mRNA hybrid
3'----TTTT----5'

Degrade RNA with alkali

3'
TTTT----5'

DNA polymerase

AAAA----3'
TTTT----5'

DNA nuclease

5'----AAAA----3' cDNA
3'----TTTT----5'

RE sticky ends

DNA ligase

RE

Plasmid DNA
vector

Recombinant
plasmid

Recombinant plasmid
enters *E. coli*

E. coli colony

cDNA library

Screen the library

Amplification

● Figure 14-6

Construction of a cDNA Library. A major disadvantage of a genomic library is that most of
the DNA fragments that are recombined with the plasmid vector are repetitive DNA sequences,
introns (noncoding regions of the gene), or spacer DNA, not DNA sequences that code for proteins. This means that the library you have to screen through to find your gene of interest (e.g.,
Factor VIII) is very large and therefore disadvantageous. The question is: Is there another way?
And the answer is: Yes, through the construction of a **complementary DNA (cDNA) library.** Please
note that the main difference between a genomic library and a cDNA library is that a genomic
library uses **genomic (chromosomal) DNA**, whereas a cDNA library uses **DNA copied from mRNA.**
DNA copied from mRNA is called cDNA. The advantage of a cDNA library should already be
apparent. In a cDNA library, you only have to screen through DNA sequences that code for proteins because the DNA used to construct the library is copied from mRNA. Because the liver synthesizes large amounts of Factor VIII, it would be a good candidate organ to use in the construction of the cDNA library. The enzyme that is critical in the formation of a cDNA library is called
reverse transcriptase. Reverse transcriptase produces DNA from an RNA template.

- All the mRNA from the liver is isolated. mRNA can be isolated by using the fact that eukaryotic
  mRNA has a poly A tail at the 3' end. A chromatograph column with oligo dT tails attached to a
  resin can be used to bind the poly A tails of the mRNA. The mRNA is then eluted off the column.
- The mRNA is hybridized with a poly (T) primer which acts as a primer for reverse transcriptase.
- Reverse transcriptase copies the mRNA into a cDNA chain, thereby forming a DNA/mRNA
  hybrid. Reverse transcriptase needs 4dNTP and magnesium for its activity.
- Alkaline conditions are used to selectively degrade the mRNA.
- DNA polymerase copies the single strand of DNA into double-stranded DNA which uses in this
  case the 3' end of the single-stranded DNA which can fold back on itself and form a few chance
  base pairings.
- A DNA nuclease cleaves the hairpin loop thus forming a double-stranded cDNA copy of the original mRNA.
- All the double-stranded cDNAs formed can be inserted into a plasmid vector to form a cDNA
  library. The cDNA has blunt ends which need to be converted to sticky ends by RE treatment to
  facilitate ligation with the plasmid.
- The cDNA library can then be screened and amplified as indicated in Figure 14-5B and C. RE =
  restriction enzyme; dNTP = deoxynucleotide triphosphate.

A

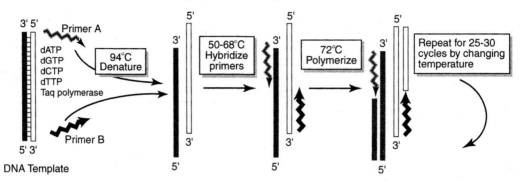

B

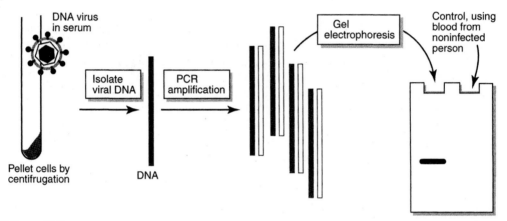

● Figure 14-7

Polymerase Chain Reaction.

In the previous discussion of cloning the Factor VIII gene using either a genomic library or cDNA library, we saw that the amplification step employed culturing bacteria in a nutrient broth overnight. There is another method to amplify DNA called polymerase chain reaction (PCR). PCR is based on **repeated cycles** of replication using **specially designed primers, DNA polymerase, dATP, dGTP, dCTP, and dTTP**. To design the primers, some knowledge of the DNA sequence to be amplified is necessary. After 20–40 repeated cycles of the PCR reaction, millions of copies of the desired DNA can be obtained within a few hours. Many PCR methods have been developed over the years as indicated below:

1. **Reverse transcription PCR (RT-PCR).** RT-PCR uses mRNA as the starting material and an initial reverse transcriptase step to produce cDNA. Eukaryotic genes contain introns (noncoding sequence) that interrupt the exons (coding sequence) and therefore will not be expressed in bacteria because bacteria do not have a splicing mechanism. So, to get a copy of a gene without introns, we can start with mRNA (the introns are already spliced out) and use RT-PCR to convert the mRNA into an intron-free DNA copy of the gene.

2. **Differential display PCR.** Differential display PCR is a type of RT-PCR that is used to compare mRNA populations from two different cell lines, tissues, or different times in embryological development to identify differentially expressed genes. This technique uses an oligo-dT primer as the first primer (because eukaryotic mRNAs have a poly A tail) and a mixture of random primers as the second primer. The PCR will produce cDNAs corresponding to all the mRNAs. The cDNAs are separated by gel electrophoresis and a series of DNA bands corresponded to all the mRNAs is displayed. The DNA bands from the different cell lines, tissues, and different times in embryological development can be compared.

3. **Real-time PCR.** Real-time PCR is a type of quantitative PCR that uses a fluorescent dye whose fluorescence increases when it binds to DNA. Because each cycle of PCR makes more DNA, the dye binds to the new DNA and the fluorescence increases. Real-time PCR uses a fluorescence-detecting thermocycler machine to amplify DNA sequences and simultaneously measure the amount of DNA produced. Most dyes do not recognize any specific DNA sequence, so these dyes just measure total DNA. However, sophisticated fluorescent probes can be constructed that recognize only a specific DNA sequence and therefore can measure a specific PCR product.

Figure 14-7A The PCR reaction:

- A region of double-stranded DNA to be amplified is shown undergoing the PCR reaction. Each cycle of the PCR reaction begins with 94°C heat treatment to separate the double-stranded DNA into single strands (denature). Because the temperature rises to 94°C, it is necessary to use **Taq polymerase** which is a thermostable DNA polymerase isolated from the thermophilic bacterium *Thermus aquaticus.* This bacterium lives in hot springs and hydrothermal vents.
- The DNA primers hybridize to the single-stranded DNA at 50–68°C.
- The DNA primers act as the primer for DNA synthesis at 72°C by DNA (Taq) polymerase, dATP, dGTP, dCTP, and dTTP.
- Of the DNA put into the original reaction, only the DNA sequence bracketed by the two primers is amplified because there are no primers attached anywhere else.
- This is repeated for 25–30 cycles to produce millions of copies of the original region of DNA.

Figure 14-7B PCR and viral detection: It is good news when a virus has been isolated and its DNA (or RNA) sequence determined because it allows one to design primers to be used in PCR. PCR is one of the most sensitive methods to detect viral infection at very early stages because of the ability of PCR to amplify DNA that is present in even very minute amounts.

- A blood sample from a suspect patient is taken and cells removed by centrifugation. If even a trace amount of virus is present in the serum, its DNA can be isolated and amplified by PCR.
- PCR will produce enough DNA so that it can be detected by gel electrophoresis.
- Note that if you want to detect an RNA virus (e.g., human immunodeficiency virus [HIV]), you must first use reverse transcriptase to convert the RNA into cDNA and then amplify by PCR.

A

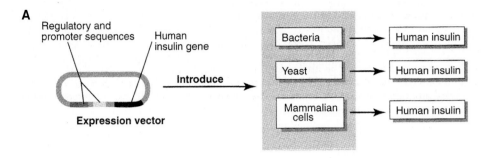

B

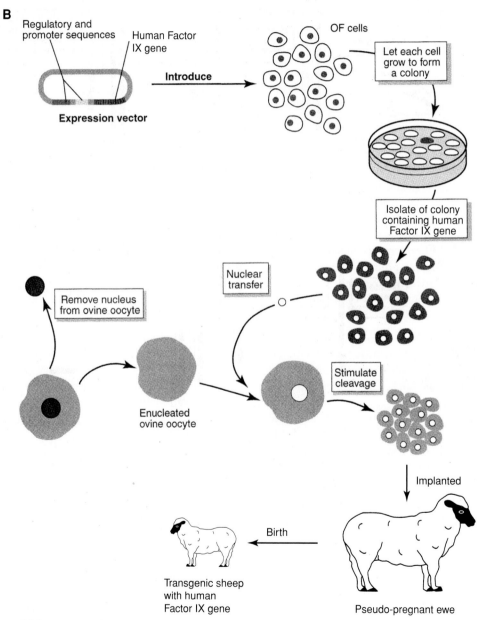

● Figure 14-8

Producing a Protein From a Cloned Gene.

We have previously discussed how a gene (e.g., Factor VIII) may be cloned using a cloning vector. After a gene has been cloned, the next step is to get the cloned gene to produce a protein, that is, be transcribed and translated into the amino acid sequence of a protein (frequently called gene expression). To do this, a plasmid vector is used (called an expression vector). Expression vectors differ from cloning vectors in that expression vectors contain gene promoter DNA sequences and gene regulatory DNA sequences that enable a nearby protein-coding DNA sequence to be expressed. Many expression vectors have been designed for use in bacteria, yeast, and mammalian cells. Expression vectors have made an important contribution to recombinant DNA technology because they allow the production of any protein (even rare proteins) in large amounts (e.g., Factor VIII, human insulin, and human growth hormone).

Figure 14-8A Expression vector. An expression vector containing regulatory and promoter DNA sequences that drive the expression of the nearby human insulin gene is shown.

- The expression vector is introduced into respective bacteria, yeast, or mammalian cells where the human insulin gene can be transcribed and translated into human insulin.
- This methodology allows for the production of large amounts of human insulin for use by all Type I and Type II diabetics in the world. This methodology has replaced the extraction of insulin from bovine pancreases collected from the slaughterhouse.

Figure 14-8B Expression vectors and nuclear transfer technique. This technique provides another method to produce large amounts of human proteins, but in this method, the human protein is produced in the **milk** of large farm animals like **transgenic sheep** or **transgenic cows. Human Factor IX** used in the treatment of **hemophilia B** has been produced in the milk of transgenic sheep. An expression vector containing regulatory and promoter DNA sequences that drive the expression of the nearby human Factor IX gene is shown.

- The expression vector is introduced into ovine fetal (OF) cells that are allowed to grow in culture to form colonies.
- The OF colony containing the human Factor IX gene is isolated.
- The nucleus is removed from one of the OF cells containing the human Factor IX gene and transferred into an enucleated ovine oocyte.
- The "new" oocyte is stimulated to undergo cleavage divisions and implanted into a pseudo-pregnant ewe.
- Transgenic sheep containing human Factor IX gene will be produced at birth. The female transgenic sheep will produce human Factor IX protein in their milk.
- Note that the nuclear transfer technique is what is giving medical bioethicists cause for grave concern because this technique leads directly to the cloning of a human being. As the nuclear transfer technique is perfected, a nucleus from one of your cells can be removed, transferred into an enucleated human oocyte, and introduced into a pseudo-pregnant woman. At birth, the offspring will be your human clone.

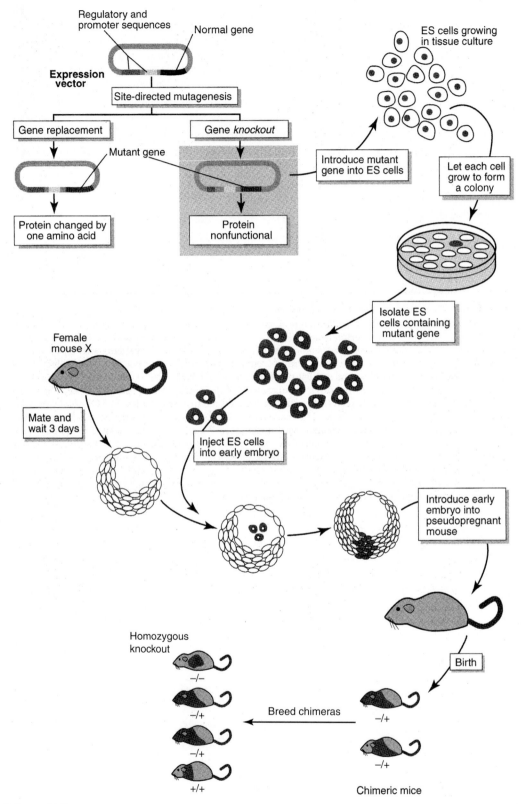

● Figure 14-9

Site-Directed Mutagenesis and Knockout Animals.
The ability to express a cloned gene within a cell opened up a new area of medical research. It is now possible to mutate a cloned gene at specific sites (called site-directed mutagenesis) and then test the function (or lack thereof) of the mutant gene. The cloned gene can be mutated so that as little as one amino acid in the protein is changed (**gene replacement**) or a large deletion can be made so that the protein is nonfunctional (called **gene knockout**). The ultimate test of the function of the mutant gene is to insert it into the genome of an animal (e.g., mouse) and observe its effect on the entire animal. A normal gene is shown in an expression vector containing regulatory and promoter DNA sequences.

- The normal gene can undergo site-directed mutagenesis so that the expressed protein is changed as little as one amino acid (gene replacement) or is rendered nonfunctional (gene knockout).
- The mutant gene within the expression vector can be introduced into embryonic stem (ES) cells.
- After culturing the ES cells, one can isolate the particular ES cells that have incorporated the mutant gene (shaded cells).
- These ES cells are then injected into an early embryo obtained from a 3-day pregnant mouse (female mouse X). This forms an early embryo containing cells from female mouse X (white cells) and ES cells with mutant gene (shaded).
- A number of these early embryos are produced and introduced to a pseudo-pregnant mouse. At birth, a number of **chimeric mice** (white and shaded areas; $-/+$) are produced. A chimeric mouse is a mouse produced from a mixture of two different cell types. Because there are two copies of every gene, the chimeric mice will have one copy of the mutant gene ($-$) and one copy of the normal gene ($+$), that is, heterozygous.
- The chimeric mice are bred and the resultant offspring will have four possibilities: $+/+$, $-/+$, $-/+$, and $-/-$. The $-/-$ homozygous knockout mouse has both copies of the gene disrupted.
- Many times, the homozygous knockout can be lethal and the mice will die before birth. Consequently, it would be ideal if we could delay turning the gene off until later in life. The **Cre-loxP recombination system** is useful in this regard.
- Cre is the C-recombination enzyme from the P1 bacteriophage and loxP is the DNA recognition site for Cre. If Cre finds two loxP sites close together, it chops out the intervening DNA and recombines the loxP sites. If the gene you wish to knockout is placed between two loxP sites, when the Cre protein is present, the gene is deleted. So, you now have an off/on switch. When Cre protein is present, the gene is off. When Cre protein is absent, the gene is on. The only question is how do you control Cre protein. This is usually done by placing the cre gene behind a promoter that can be directly controlled in an experimental situation or behind a promoter of a gene that is expressed under some experimental condition we can control.

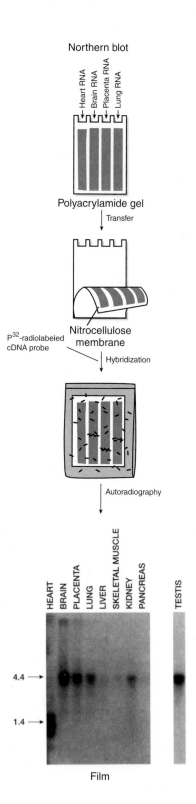

Northern Blot (mRNA):

- A Northern blot is a variant of a Southern blot that separates undigested **mRNA** based on size by PAGE.
- A Northern blot is used to determine whether a gene is being expressed or not within a certain tissue by analyzing **mRNA levels.**
- The variable-sized mRNAs are transferred to nitrocellulose membrane and then hybridized with a radiolabeled P^{32} **cDNA probe.** The P^{32} cDNA probe is identical to the **template DNA strand** that produced the mRNA.
- Photographic film is then placed over the nitrocellulose membrane, exposed, and developed (autoradiography).
- Radiolabeled cDNA probe hybridization to specific mRNAs is documented by dark bands on the photographic film.
- A real Northern blot using a radiolabeled cDNA probe for the **FMR1 gene** (Fragile X mental retardation syndrome). Note that the highest levels of mRNA coded by the *FMR1* gene are found in the brain and testes (4.4 kb). Smaller transcripts of the mRNA (1.4 kb) are found in the heart. This means that the *FMR1* gene is expressed most highly in the brain and testes.

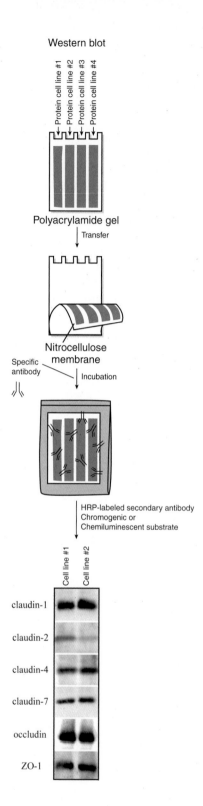

Western Blot (Protein):

- A Western blot separates **proteins** from various cell lines (1–4) based on size by PAGE.
- The proteins are transferred to a nitrocellulose membrane and then incubated with an antibody to a specific protein.
- Antibody binding to specific proteins may be detected by a **horseradish peroxidase (HRP)–labeled secondary antibody** which can be reacted with a **chromogenic substrate** (usually brown in color).
- A recent improvement in the technique uses a **chemiluminescent substrate**. In this case, antibody binding to specific proteins may be detected by an HRP–labeled secondary antibody which can be reacted with a chemiluminescent substrate. The chemiluminescent substrate allows detection sensitivities superior to that of a chromogenic substrate, whereby picogram protein levels of detection can be achieved using either X-ray film or imaging equipment.
- Antibody binding to specific proteins is documented by colored bands on the nitrocellulose membrane (using a chromogenic substrate shown) or X-ray film (using a chemiluminescent substrate not shown).
- A real Western blot shows a composite of six different Western blots for two different cell lines (1 and 2). Antibody binding to specific proteins (i.e., claudin-1, claudin-2, claudin-4, claudin-7, occludin, and ZO-1) is detected by an HRP and a chromogenic substrate. Note that the expression of the proteins is similar in both cell line 1 and cell line 2, except that claudin-2 appears to be more highly expressed in cell line 1 than in cell line 2.
- **Positively charged histone proteins.** In general, most proteins are negatively charged and therefore can be separated using "normal" SDS-PAGE conditions which produce anionic SDS-protein complexes. However, histones are **positively charged** and therefore Acid-Urea-PAGE conditions are used to run positively charged proteins such as histones. Urea keeps the histones from forming aggregates. In addition, the electric field needs to be reversed so that the positively charged histones will migrate toward the bottom of the gel.

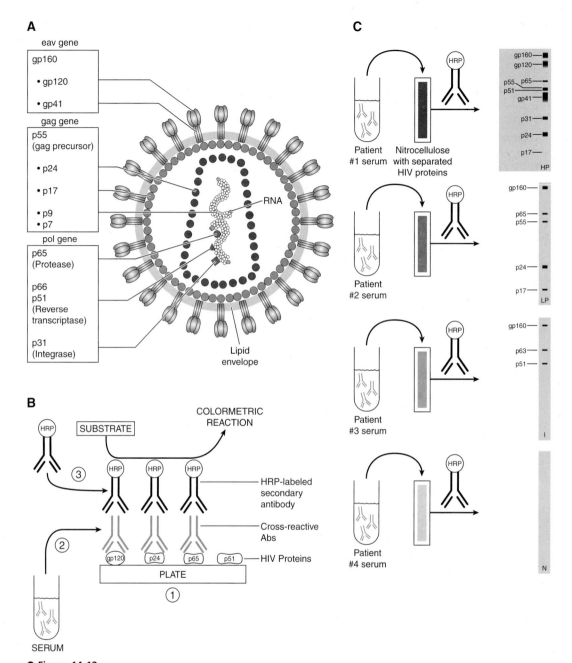

● Figure 14-12

Human Immunodeficiency Virus (HIV) Structure:

- HIV belonging to the *Retroviridae* family and *Lentivirinae* subfamily is a nonsegmented, single-stranded, diploid (two identical strands of the RNA genome), positive sense RNA (ss+ RNA) virus. The following HIV genes are important in HIV testing:
  - The *env* gene which encodes for
    - gp160 (an envelope glycoprotein which is later cleaved into gp120 and gp41)
    - gp120 (binds to the CD4 receptor protein)
    - gp41 (a transmembrane protein)
  - The *gag* gene (group-specific antigen) which encodes for
    - p55 (the gag precursor protein)
    - p24 (capsid protein)
    - p17 (matrix protein)
    - p9 (nucleocapsid protein)
    - p7 (nucleocapsid protein)
  - The *pol* gene which encodes for
    - p65 (a protease)
    - p66 and p51 (reverse transcriptase dimer)
    - p31 (integrase)

   Figure 14-12B HIV ELISA (enzyme-linked immunoabsorbent assay) test. The serologic tests for HIV infection are based upon detection of **antibodies in the serum directed against HIV proteins.** The ELISA is the first test used clinically to detect the possibility of HIV infection. Remember that the ELISA does NOT detect the HIV virus per se but only antibodies directed against HIV proteins. The HIV ELISA test can produce **false-positive results** which means that a person's serum may contain cross-reactive antibodies to HIV proteins even though the person has never been exposed to HIV. Sources of false positives include multiple pregnancies, multiple blood transfusions, autoimmune disorders, chronic hepatitis, chronic alcoholism, hepatitis B vaccination, influenza vaccination, rabies vaccination, renal failure, cystic fibrosis, syphilis infection, malaria infection (important because many Africans are exposed to malaria), infection with other human retroviruses (e.g., HTLV 1/II), association with large animals (e.g., animal trainers, veterinarians), and hemodialysis. An ELISA includes the following steps:

- A number of known HIV proteins are attached to a plate
- A person's serum is applied to the plate. If the person's serum has antibodies (Abs) that cross-react with HIV proteins, the antibodies will bind to the HIV proteins.
- Antibody binding to HIV proteins can be detected by an HRP-labeled secondary antibody which can be reacted with a chromogenic substrate to produce a colormetric reaction (usually brown in color).

   Figure 14-12C HIV Western blot test. If a positive ELISA result is obtained, it must be confirmed by a Western blot. Again, remember that an HIV Western blot does NOT detect the HIV virus per se but only antibodies directed against HIV proteins.

- A number of known HIV proteins are separated based on size by PAGE. The separated HIV proteins are transferred to a nitrocellulose membrane. A person's serum is applied to the nitrocellulose membrane. If the person's serum has antibodies (Abs) that cross-react with HIV proteins, the antibodies will bind to the HIV proteins. Antibody binding to HIV proteins can be detected by an HRP-labeled secondary antibody which can be reacted with a chromogenic substrate to produce a colormetric reaction (usually brown in color).
- Patient no. 1 shows a high positive (HP) HIV Western blot reaction.
- Patient no. 2 shows a low positive (LP) HIV Western blot reaction.
- Patient no. 3 shows an indeterminate (I) HIV Western blot reaction. Almost all HIV-infected patients with an indeterminate result will develop a positive result within 1 month (called seroconversion).
- Patient no. 4 shows a negative (N) result.

   To identify the actual HIV virus, **nucleic acid-based tests** (e.g., RT-PCR, Quantiplex branched DNA test) are used to detect a 142-base target sequence in a highly conserved region of the HIV *gag* gene. These tests use a patient's **white blood cells** because retroviruses incorporate into host cell DNA. These tests are not used in population screening but generally later in the disease process to assess the **viral load** in an AIDS patient undergoing antiretroviral drug therapy.

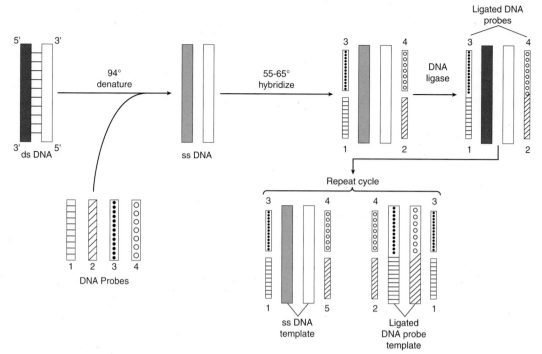

● **Figure 14-13**

Ligase Chain Reaction (LCR).

LCR is a DNA amplification technique that detects specific DNA sequences by amplifying the DNA probes. LCR can be used to identify tumor types, to detect single-base mutation genetic disorders (e.g., sickle cell disease), and to detect infectious diseases (e.g., *Chlamydia trachomatis*, gonorrhea). LCR involves the following steps:

- Each cycle of the LCR reaction begins with 94°C heat treatment to separate the double-stranded DNA (dsDNA) into single-stranded DNA (ssDNA), that is, denatured.
- The DNA probes include four probes (nos. 1, 2, 3, 4) one for every side of the ssDNA. The DNA probes hybridize to the ssDNA at 55–65°C.
- As long as there are no base mismatches at the junction of the DNA probes, DNA ligase can ligate each pair of DNA probes to form ligated DNA probes.
- The cycle is repeated, whereby both ssDNA and the ligated DNA probes are used as templates. The ability of ligated DNA probes to serve as templates in subsequent cycles leads to exponential amplification.

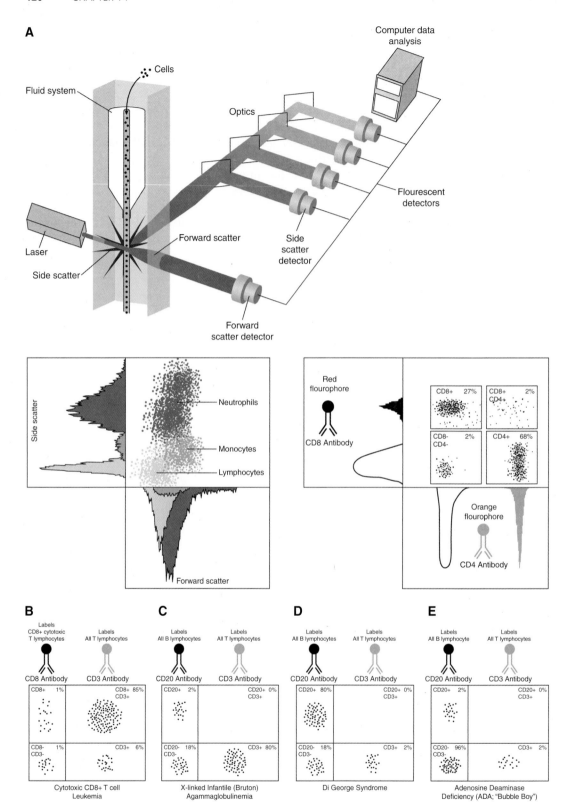

● Figure 14-14

Flow Cytometry.

Flow cytometry is a technique for the analysis of multiple parameters of cells within a heterogenous population. Parameters include cell size, intracellular complexity (granules, nucleus shape, etc.), and cell surface fluorescent staining.

- The fluidic system passes thousands of cells per second through a laser beam one at a time.
- As the cell passes through the laser, the cell will scatter light in the **forward direction** called **forward scatter.** The forward scatter light is quantified by a detector which converts the light intensity into a voltage pulse. The size of the voltage pulse recorded for each cell that passes through the laser is proportional to **cell size. Therefore, forward scatter allows the measurement of cell size.** This data is plotted on a histogram.
- As the cell passes through the laser, the cell will also scatter light in the side direction called **side scatter.** The side scatter light is quantified by a detector (located 90 degrees to the laser path) which again converts the light intensity into a voltage pulse. The size of the voltage pulse recorded for each cell that passes through the laser is proportional to **intracellular complexity. Therefore, side scatter allows the identification of intracellular complexity.** This data is plotted on a histogram.
- The histograms of the forward scatter (X axis) and side scatter (Y axis) can be combined to form a **two-dimensional dot plot.** A two-dimensional dot plot of flow cytometry using peripheral blood shows three populations: lymphocytes, monocytes, and neutrophils. **Remember that each dot on a dot plot represents a cell.**
- A common method used to study cell characteristics using flow cytometry involves the use of fluorescent-labeled antibodies that bind to the cell surface. When a fluorescent-labeled cell passes through the laser, the laser will strike the fluorophore and a fluorescent signal will be emitted. The fluorescent signal is quantified by a detector which converts the fluorescence intensity into a voltage pulse. The size of the voltage pulse recorded for each cell that passes through the laser is proportional to the **amount of fluorescence emitted.**
- A typical flow cytometry study uses two fluorescent-labeled antibodies. For example, a CD8 antibody with a red fluorophore identifies $CD8^+$ T lymphocytes and a CD4 antibody with an orange fluorophore identifies $CD4^+$ T lymphocytes. The data for each antibody is plotted on a histogram. The histograms can be combined to form a two-dimensional dot plot. A two-dimensional dot plot of this example studying T lymphocytes in peripheral blood shows four populations: a $CD8^+$ T lymphocytes making up ~27% of the cells, $CD8^+$ and $CD4^+$ T lymphocytes making up ~2% of the cells, $CD8^-$ and $CD4^-$ T lymphocytes making up ~2% of the cells, and $CD4^+$ T lymphocytes making up ~68% of the cells.

Figure 14-14B Two-dimensional dot plot of a cytotoxic $CD8^+$ T-cell leukemia. Peripheral blood sample from a leukemia patient is run through flow cytometry using two fluorescent-labeled antibodies: CD8 antibody which labels $CD8^+$ cytotoxic T lymphocytes and CD3 antibody which labels all T lymphocytes. The two-dimensional dot plot shows four populations of cells with $CD8^+$ and $CD3^+$ T lymphocytes making up 85% of the cells. This high percentage (85%) would be consistent with a cytotoxic $CD8^+$ T-cell leukemia where the patient has a **large increase in $CD8^+$ cytotoxic T lymphocytes.**

Figure 14-14C Two-dimensional dot plot of X-linked infantile (Bruton) agammaglobulinemia. Peripheral blood sample from a patient is run through flow cytometry using two fluorescent-labeled antibodies: CD20 antibody which labels all B lymphocytes and CD3 antibody which labels all T lymphocytes. The two-dimensional dot plot shows four populations of cells with $CD20^+$ B lymphocytes making up only 2% of the cells and $CD3^+$ T lymphocytes making up 80% of the cells. These percentages would be consistent with X-linked infantile (Bruton) agammaglobulinemia where the patient basically has **no B lymphocytes but only T lymphocytes present.** Note that there can never be any $CD20^+$ and $CD3^+$ cells because these two markers have been chosen to distinguish B lymphocytes from T lymphocytes; there can never be a B lymphocyte that is also $CD3^+$, and visa versa.

Figure 14-14D Two-dimensional dot plot of DiGeorge syndrome. Peripheral blood sample from a patient is run through flow cytometry using two fluorescent-labeled antibodies: CD20 antibody which labels all B lymphocytes and CD3 antibody which labels all T lymphocytes. The two-dimensional dot plot shows four populations of cells with $CD20^+$ B lymphocytes making up 80%

of the cells and CD3$^+$ T lymphocytes making up 2% of the cells. These percentages would be consistent with DiGeorge syndrome where the patient basically **has B lymphocytes but no T lymphocytes.**

Figure 14-14E Two-dimensional dot plot of adenosine deaminase deficiency (ADA; "Bubble Boy"). Peripheral blood sample from a patient is run through flow cytometry using two fluorescent-labeled antibodies: CD20 antibody which labels all B lymphocytes and CD3 antibody which labels all T lymphocytes. The two-dimensional dot plot shows four populations of cells with CD 20$^+$ B lymphocytes making up only 2% of the cells and CD3$^+$ T lymphocytes making up only 2% of the cells. These percentages would be consistent with ADA ("Bubble Boy") where the patient basically has **no B lymphocytes and T lymphocytes.**

Chapter 15

Identification of Human Disease Genes

I **General Features.** There is no one particular way that a human gene involved in a disease is identified. Molecular biologists use a large variety of molecular techniques to investigate each situation on a case-by-case basis.

II **Identification of a Human Disease Gene Through a Chromosome Abnormality**

A. **SOTOS SYNDROME** (also called **Cerebral Gigantism; Figure 15-1**). Sotos syndrome is a syndrome found in infants that tend to be large at birth and continue to grow rapidly during the early years of childhood. Clinical findings include macrocephaly, high forehead, frontal bossing, downward slanting of palpebral fissures, hypertelorism, prominent jaw, sparse hair in frontoparietal region, high arched palate, mental retardation, and poor coordination.

B. A Sotos patient was found with a chromosome translocation between band q35 on chromosome 5 and band q24 on chromosome 8, t(5;8)(q35;q24).

C. The DNA from this patient was isolated and inserted into various cloning vectors (e.g., cosmids, bacterial artificial chromosomes, and Plasmid artificial chromosomes).

D. Clones containing the breakpoint were identified by FISH (fluorescence in situ hybridization) and the DNA sequencing around the breakpoint was done.

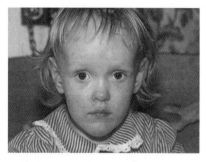

● Figure 15-1 Sotos Syndrome.

E. The DNA sequence was found to be a homologue of the **mouse Nsd1 gene** by computer analysis of gene databases.

F. Subsequently, a human genomic library was screened using a DNA probe constructed from the mouse Nsd1 gene, and the **human NSD1 gene** on chromosome 5q35 was cloned.

G. Once the NSD1 gene was cloned, DNA from other Sotos patients was analyzed and mutations and/or microdeletions in the NSD1 gene were found.

H. This confirmed that mutations and/or microdeletions in the NSD1 gene are directly involved in the Sotos syndrome. The NSD1 gene encodes for the **NSD1 protein** (<u>n</u>uclear <u>r</u>eceptor binding <u>SET</u> <u>d</u>omain protein <u>1</u>) which is a **histone methyltransferase** that acts as a transcriptional intermediary factor capable of negatively and positively influencing transcription. Figure 15-1 shows a young girl with Sotos syndrome.

III   # Identification of a Human Disease Gene Through Pure Transcript Mapping

A. TREACHER COLLINS FRANCESCHETTI SYNDROME (TCOF; Figure 15-2). A First Arch syndrome results from abnormal development of **pharyngeal arch 1** and produces various facial anomalies. First Arch syndromes are caused by a lack of migration of **neural crest cells** into pharyngeal arch 1. A well-described First Arch syndrome is the TCOF syndrome. TCOF is an autosomal dominant genetic disorder caused by a mutation in the *TCOFI* gene on **chromosome 5q32–33.1** for the **treacle protein**. Clinical findings include hypoplasia of the zygomatic bones and mandible resulting in midface hypoplasia, micrognathia, and retrognathia; external ear abnormalities including small, absent, malformed, or rotated ears; and lower eyelid abnormalities including coloboma.

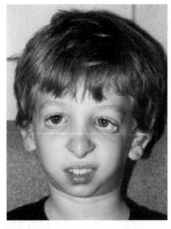

● **Figure 15-2 Treacher Collins Franceschetti Syndrome.**

B. Genetic linkage studies established linkage to markers on **chromosome 5q32–33.1**. The purpose of genetic linkage is to identify a crude chromosomal location of a particular gene locus or gene allele. Genetic loci on the same chromosome that are physically close to one another tend to stay together during meiosis in germ cells and are thus **genetically linked**. Recombination occurs in germ cells during meiosis. As recombination occurs, if there is a large physical distance between two gene loci, there is a good chance that crossover will occur between them and the two gene loci will not stay together and therefore segregate independently among the gametes. However, if there is a small physical distance between two gene loci, there is a good chance that crossover will <u>not</u> occur between them and the two gene loci will stay together and therefore segregate together among the gametes. In genetic linkage studies, disease genes are mapped by measuring recombination against a panel of different markers spread over the entire genome.

C. A YAC **clone contig** for chromosome 5q32–33.1 was constructed. A number of genes were identified in this region. A clone contig is one of a set of overlapping clones that represent a continuous region of DNA. More genetic linkage studies eventually produced a candidate gene called the *TCOF1* gene.

D. The *TCOF1* gene showed no homologous relationship to any other gene by computer analysis of gene databases.

E. DNA from other TCOF patients was analyzed and mutations and/or microdeletions in the TCOF1 gene were found.

F. This confirmed that mutations and/or microdeletions in the human *TCOF1* gene are directly involved in the TCOF syndrome. The *TCOF1* gene encodes for the **treacle protein** which is a nucleolar protein related to the nucleolar phosphoprotein **Nopp140** both of which contain **LIS1 motifs** leading to the speculation of **microtubule dynamics** involvement. In addition, treacle protein interacts with the small nucleolar ribonucleoprotein **hNop56p** leading to the speculation of **ribosomal biogenesis** involvement. Figure 15-2 shows a young boy with TCOF syndrome.

IV Identification of a Human Disease Gene Through Large Scale DNA Sequencing

A. **BRANCHIO-OTO-RENAL SYNDROME (BOR SYNDROME; Figure 15-3).** External ear malformations and renal anomalies occur in several multiple congenital anomaly syndromes (e.g., BOR syndrome, CHARGE association, Townes-Brocks syndrome, Nager syndrome, Miller syndrome, and diabetic embryopathy). The BOR syndrome is an autosomal dominant genetic disorder found in infants. Clinical findings include pharyngeal fistulas along the side of the neck, malformation of the external and internal ear, hearing loss, hypoplasia, or absence of the kidneys.

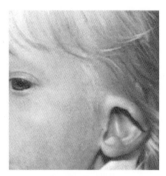

● Figure 15-3 Branchio-Oto-Renal Syndrome.

B. A BOR patient was found with a rearrangement of chromosome 8q13.

C. A PAC clone contig for a region around 8q13 was constructed.

D. Large scale DNA sequencing of the 8q13 region was done.

E. The DNA sequence was found to be a homologue of the **Drosophila *Eya* gene** (eyes absent) by computer analysis of gene databases.

F. Subsequently, a cDNA library using 9-week total fetal mRNA was screened using a DNA probe constructed from the Drosophila *Eya* gene, and the **human *EYA1* gene** was cloned.

G. Once the *EYA1* gene was cloned, DNA from other BOR patients was analyzed and mutations and/or microdeletions in the *EYA1* gene were found. This confirmed that mutations and/or microdeletions in the human EYA1 gene are directly involved in the BOR syndrome. The *EYA1* gene encodes for the **EYA1 protein** (**e**yes **a**bsent homolog 1 protein) which has intrinsic phosphatase activity enabling it to serve as a promoter-specific **transcriptional coactivator.** EYA1 protein interacts with several other proteins, including SIX1 and SIX5, to regulate the activity of genes involved in many aspects of embryonic development. Figure 15-3 shows a young girl with an ear malformation typical of BOR syndrome.

Ⓥ Identification of a Human Disease Gene Through Comparison of Human and Mouse Maps

A. WAARDENBURG SYNDROME TYPE 1 (WS1; Figure 15-4). WS1 is an autosomal dominant genetic disorder caused by mutation in the *PAX3* gene on **chromosome 2q35** for the **PAX3 paired box protein.** The *PAX* genes are characterized by a 128 amino acid DNA-binding domain called a paired box. Clinical findings include dystopia canthorum (lateral displacement of the inner canthi), growing together of eyebrows, lateral displacement of lacrimal puncta, a broad nasal root, heterochromia of the iris, congenital deafness or hearing impairment, and piebaldism including a white forelock and a triangular area of hypopigmentation.

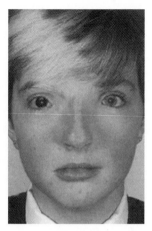

● **Figure 15-4 Waardenburg Syndrome Type 1.**

B. Genetic linkage studies established linkage to markers on human chromosome 2q. The human chromosome 2q region has strong synteny (i.e., general correspondence) to a portion of mouse chromosome 1.

C. A mouse mutant called the **Splotch (Sp) mutant** was described with pigmentary abnormalities due to the patchy absence of melanocytes. The phenotypic similarities between WS Type 1 and the Splotch mutant mouse suggested that homologous genes were involved. The **mouse *Pax-3* gene** was linked to the Splotch mutant.

D. Subsequently, a human genomic library was screened using a DNA probe constructed from the mouse *Pax-3* gene, and the **human *PAX3* gene** was cloned.

E. Once the *PAX3* gene was cloned, DNA from other WS Type 1 patients was analyzed, and mutations and/or microdeletions in the *PAX3* gene were found. This confirmed that mutations and/or microdeletions in the human *PAX3* gene are directly involved in the WS Type 1 syndrome. The *PAX3* gene encodes for the **PAX3 protein (paired box protein 3)** which is a **DNA-binding transcription factor** that is expressed in the early embryo and regulates neural crest-derived cell types, including melanocytes. Figure 15-4 shows a teenage boy with Waardenburg syndrome.

Chapter 16

Gene Therapy

1 Gene Therapy. Gene therapy involves the genetic modification of a patient's cells to achieve a positive therapeutic outcome. There are two types of gene therapy as indicated below.

A. GERM-LINE GENE THERAPY

1. Germ-line gene therapy involves the genetic modification of a **gamete, zygote, or a preimplantation embryo** that produces a permanent modification that can be transmitted to other generations.

2. Germ-line gene therapy is not a realistic option at present for purely technical reasons, but there are also serious ethical questions that have resulted in this type of gene therapy being prohibited by law in many countries.

B. SOMATIC CELL GENE THERAPY. Somatic cell gene therapy involves the genetic modification of specific **somatic cells or tissues** of a particular patient. All current gene therapy clinical trials and protocols are for somatic cell gene therapy. There are a number of novel approaches to somatic cell gene therapy which include the following:

1. **Gene augmentation**
   a. This approach involves the insertion of a **functioning copy of a gene** into a diseased somatic cell or tissue to express a curative protein.
   b. This approach is used to treat a **loss-of-function mutation**.

2. **Inhibition of gene expression**
   a. This approach involves the insertion of **microRNA (miRNA) or small interfering RNA (siRNA); antisense RNA; or ribozyme** into a diseased somatic cell of tissue to block expression of a certain mutated gene.
   b. This approach is used to treat a **gain-of-function mutation**.
   c. miRNA can inhibit the translation of a complementary mRNA by forming dsRNA which either physically blocks mRNA translation or is degraded by RNA-Induced Silencing *Complex*, or *RISC*.
   d. **Antisense RNA** can inhibit the translation of a complementary mRNA by forming dsRNA which either physically blocks mRNA translation or is degraded by **RNAse H**. Antisense RNA therapy has rather unpredictable results, where the translation of the target gene may be silenced efficiently; nonspecific effects; or little-to-no effect.
   e. **Ribozyme** (e.g., hammerhead, hairpin, human delta virus, Varkud satellite) is an RNA molecule that has enzymatic activity to degrade mRNA. A ribozyme can be designed to bind to a complementary mRNA and then degrade the mRNA.

3. **Direct killing of disease cells.** This approach involves the insertion of a **prodrug gene** into a diseased somatic cell or tissue to express a curative drug.

4. **Assisted killing of disease cells.** This approach involves the insertion of a **foreign antigen gene** into the diseased somatic cell or tissue to stimulate an immune response against the diseased cells.

Ⅱ Ex Vivo and In Vivo Gene Therapy

A. EX VIVO GENE THERAPY involves the removal a patient's cells (e.g., hematopoietic cells, skin cells), insertion of a therapeutic gene, amplification of the genetically modified cells in culture, and return of the genetically modified cells to the patient. Ex vivo gene therapy is only applicable to cells that can be easily removed from and returned to the patient.

B. IN VIVO GENE THERAPY involves the insertion of a therapeutic gene directly into a patient's tissue (e.g., muscle) or directly into the general circulation but designed so that the therapeutic gene is directed to only the desired cell or tissue.

Ⅲ Integration into Host Cell Chromosomes or as Episomes

A. HOST CELL CHROMOSOMES

1. The insertion of the therapeutic gene into the host cell chromosomes will result in the replication of the therapeutic gene whenever the host cell divides. This results in **long-term expression** of the therapeutic gene but with serious risks.

2. Because the insertion of the therapeutic gene into the host cell chromosomes is a random event, a number of less-than advantageous possibilities exist which include as follows:

   a. The therapeutic gene may **never be expressed, expressed at low levels,** or **expressed for a short time and then silenced.**

   b. The therapeutic gene may insert within the DNA sequence of a normal gene and inactivate the normal gene.

   c. The therapeutic gene may activate a nearby proto-oncogene leading to cancer (*Note*: this occurred in two children who underwent gene therapy for severe combined immunodeficiency and later develop a novel type of T-cell leukemia).

B. EPISOMES

1. The insertion of the therapeutic gene as extrachromosomal episomes will not result in the replication of the therapeutic gene whenever the host cell divides. This results in **short-term expression** of the therapeutic gene because the episomes will be diluted out as the cell population grows.

2. This means that repeated treatments may be necessary, but the safety of a self-limiting process will likely make this a mainstay therapy tool.

Ⅳ Viral Vectors Used in Gene Therapy. Most protocols for human gene therapy employ the use of a wide variety of mammalian viruses as vectors which are designed to include a therapeutic gene. These vectors include the following:

A. ONCORETROVIRAL VECTORS

1. The oncoretroviruses are **RNA viruses** that deliver a nucleoprotein complex into the **cytoplasm of the cell.**

2. The viral RNA genome is transcribed using **reverse transcriptase** into cDNA.

3. The cDNA is then used as a template to make a second strand forming dsDNA.

4. The dsDNA is inserted into the **host cell chromosomes.**

5. The dsDNA gains access to the host cell chromosomes only during mitosis when the nuclear envelope disintegrates. This means that oncoretroviral vectors can be used **only in dividing cells.**

B. ADENOVIRAL VECTORS

1. The adenoviruses are **dsDNA viruses** that deliver their DNA genome into the **nucleus of the cell**. The dsDNA remains in the nucleus as an **episome**.

2. The viral DNA gains access to the nucleus in both **dividing and nondividing cells**.

3. The major problem with adenoviral vectors is the occurrence of **unwanted immune reactions** in the patient (e.g., a gene therapy trial for **ornithine transcarbamylase deficiency** resulted in the death of the patient 2 days after receiving an intrahepatic injection of an adenoviral vectors containing a therapeutic gene).

4. In addition, episomes result in the **short-term expression** of the therapeutic gene (e.g., a gene therapy trial for **cystic fibrosis** resulted in a decline in expression of the therapeutic gene after 2 weeks and no expression after 4 weeks).

C. ADENO-ASSOCIATED VIRUS VECTORS (AVAs)

1. The AVAs are **single-stranded DNA viruses** that rely on coinfection by an adenovirus or herpes helper virus to replicate.

2. The DNA gets inserted into a specific site at **host cell chromosome 19q13.3** which is a highly desirable property because it eliminates many of less than advantageous possibilities connected to integration into host cell chromosomes (see IIIA2 above).

3. The major problem with AVAs is that they are small and can accommodate **inserts of only ≈4.5 kb.**

D. LENTIVIRUS VECTORS

1. The lentiviruses are **RNA viruses** that deliver a nucleoprotein complex into the **cytoplasm of the cell**.

2. The viral RNA genome is transcribed using **reverse transcriptase** into cDNA.

3. The cDNA is then used as a template to make a second strand forming dsDNA.

4. dsDNA is inserted into the **host cell chromosomes**.

5. Unlike oncoretroviral vectors, the dsDNA gains access to the host cell chromosomes in **nondividing cells**.

6. The most popular lentivirus used to construct lentivirus vectors is the **human immunodeficiency virus** which understandably causes great concern for inadvertently generating a competent virus.

E. HERPES SIMPLEX VIRUS VECTORS

1. The herpes simplex viruses are **dsDNA viruses** that are tropic for the central nervous system and can establish a lifelong latent infection in sensory ganglia.

2. The dsDNA remains in the nucleus as an **episome**.

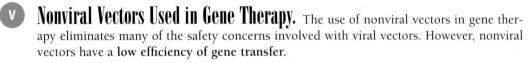

V Nonviral Vectors Used in Gene Therapy. The use of nonviral vectors in gene therapy eliminates many of the safety concerns involved with viral vectors. However, nonviral vectors have a **low efficiency of gene transfer**.

A. LIPOSOMES

1. Liposomes are **synthetic lipid vesicles**.

2. Cationic liposomes form with DNA bound on the outside of the liposome and anionic liposomes form with DNA bound in the inside of the liposome.

3. The liposomes bind to the cell membrane and then allow the DNA to enter the **cytoplasm of the cell**.

4. Most gene therapy protocols use cationic liposomes.

5. The DNA inserted into the cell remains as an **episome**.

B. DIRECT INJECTION

1. DNA can be injected directly with a needle and syringe (e.g., in muscle tissue for gene therapy of Duchenne muscular dystrophy).

2. The DNA inserted into the cell remains as an **episome**.

C. RECEPTOR-MEDIATED ENDOCYTOSIS

1. The DNA is coupled to a targeting molecule (e.g., asialoglycoprotein or transferrin) that binds to specific cell membrane receptors (e.g., asialoglycoprotein receptors on hepatocytes or transferrin receptors on hematopoietic cells).
2. The binding to a specific cell membrane receptor induces receptor-mediated endocytosis and transfer of DNA into the **cytoplasm of the cell**.
3. In general, substances internalized by receptor-mediated endocytosis are directed to **endolysosomes** for degradation. Therefore, the vector must be designed with some mechanism to allow for **escape from lysosomal degradation** (e.g., cotransfer with an adenovirus which disrupts the endolysosome and allows escape).
4. The DNA inserted into the cell remains as an **episome**.

The Genetic Code

1st Position (5' end)	2nd Position				3rd Position (3' end)
	U	C	A	G	
U	Phe	Ser	Tyr	Cys	U
	Phe	Ser	Tyr	Cys	C
	Leu	Ser	**STOP**	**STOP**	A
	Leu	Ser	**STOP**	Trp	G
C	Leu	Pro	His	Arg	U
	Leu	Pro	His	Arg	C
	Leu	Pro	Gln	Arg	A
	Leu	Pro	Gln	Arg	G
A	Ile	Thr	Asn	Ser	U
	Ile	Thr	Asn	Ser	C
	Ile	Thr	Lys	Arg	A
	Met	Thr	Lys	Arg	G
G	Val	Ala	Asp	Gly	U
	Val	Ala	Asp	Gly	C
	Val	Ala	Glu	Gly	A
	Val	Ala	Glu	Gly	G

Amino Acids

Amino Acids			Codons
A	Ala	Alanine	GCA GCC GCG GCU
C	Cys	Cysteine	UGC UGC
D	Asp	Aspartic acid	GAC GAU
E	Glu	Glutamic acid	GAA GAG
F	Phe	Phenylalanine	UUC UUU
G	Gly	Glycine	GGA GGC GGG GGU
H	His	Histidine	CAC CAU
I	Ile	Isoleucine	AUA AUC AUU
K	Lys	Lysine	AAA AAG
L	Leu	Leucine	UUA UUG CUA CUC CUG CUU
M	Met	Methionine	AUG
N	Asn	Asparagine	AAC AAAU
P	Pro	Proline	CCA CCC CCG CCU
Q	Gln	Glutamine	CAA CAG
R	Arg	Arginine	AGA AGG CGA CGC CGG CGU
S	Ser	Serine	AGC AGU UCA UCC UCG UCU
T	Thr	Threonine	ACA ACC ACG ACU
V	Val	Valine	GUA GUC GUG GUU
W	Trp	Tryptophan	UGG
Y	Tyr	Tyrosine	UAC UAU

Chromosomal Locations of Human Genetic Diseases

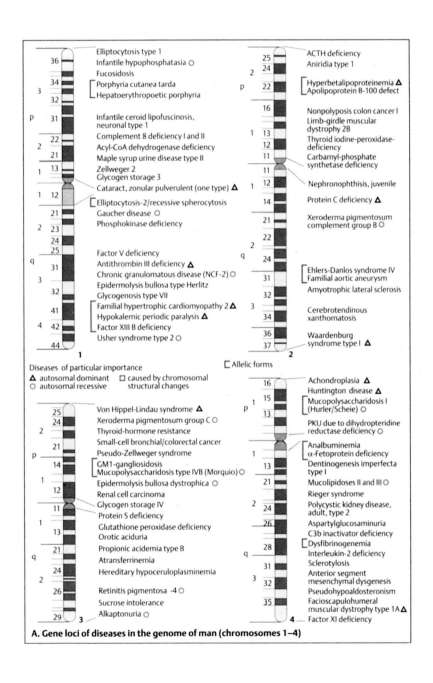

A. Gene loci of diseases in the genome of man (chromosomes 1–4)

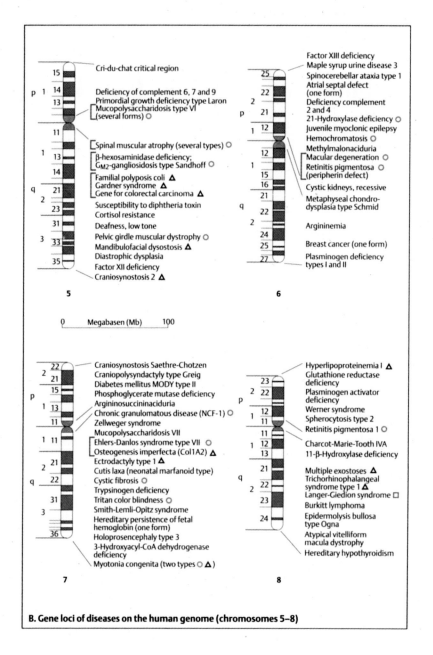

B. Gene loci of diseases on the human genome (chromosomes 5–8)

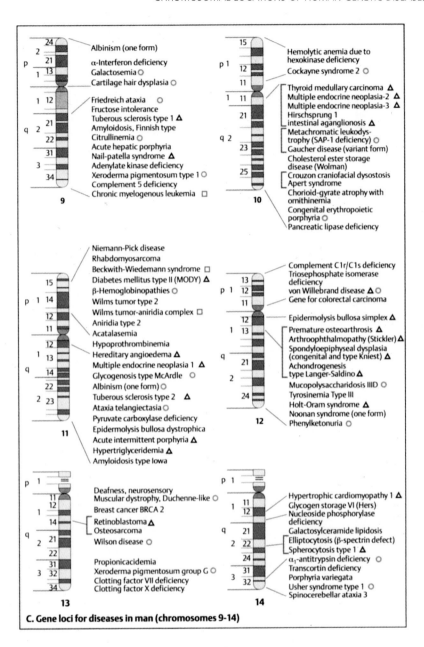

Chromosome 9
- Albinism (one form)
- α-Interferon deficiency
- Galactosemia ○
- Cartilage hair dysplasia ○
- Friedreich ataxia ○
- Fructose intolerance
- Tuberous sclerosis type 1 △
- Amyloidosis, Finnish type
- Citrullinemia ○
- Acute hepatic porphyria
- Nail-patella syndrome △
- Adenylate kinase deficiency
- Xeroderma pigmentosum type 1 ○
- Complement 5 deficiency
- Chronic myelogenous leukemia □

Chromosome 10
- Hemolytic anemia due to hexokinase deficiency
- Cockayne syndrome 2 ○
- Thyroid medullary carcinoma △
- Multiple endocrine neoplasia-2 △
- Multiple endocrine neoplasia-3 △
- Hirschsprung 1 intestinal aganglionosis △
- Metachromatic leukodystrophy (SAP-1 deficiency) ○
- Gaucher disease (variant form)
- Cholesterol ester storage disease (Wolman)
- Crouzon craniofacial dysostosis
- Apert syndrome
- Chorioid-gyrate atrophy with ornithinemia
- Congenital erythropoietic porphyria ○
- Pancreatic lipase deficiency

Chromosome 11
- Niemann-Pick disease
- Rhabdomyosarcoma
- Beckwith-Wiedemann syndrome □
- Diabetes mellitus type II (MODY) △
- β-Hemoglobinopathies ○
- Wilms tumor type 2
- Wilms tumor-aniridia complex □
- Aniridia type 2
- Acatalasemia
- Hypoprothrombinemia
- Hereditary angioedema △
- Multiple endocrine neoplasia 1 △
- Glycogenosis type McArdle ○
- Albinism (one form) ○
- Tuberous sclerosis type 2 △
- Ataxia telangiectasia ○
- Pyruvate carboxylase deficiency
- Epidermolysis bullosa dystrophica
- Acute intermittent porphyria △
- Hypertriglyceridemia △
- Amyloidosis type Iowa

Chromosome 12
- Complement C1r/C1s deficiency
- Triosephosphate isomerase deficiency
- von Willebrand disease △ ○
- Gene for colorectal carcinoma
- Epidermolysis bullosa simplex △
- Premature osteoarthrosis △
- Arthroophthalmopathy (Stickler) △
- Spondyloepiphyseal dysplasia (congenital and type Kniest) △
- Achondrogenesis type Langer-Saldino △
- Mucopolysaccharidosis IIID ○
- Tyrosinemia Type III
- Holt-Oram syndrome △
- Noonan syndrome (one form)
- Phenylketonuria ○

Chromosome 13
- Deafness, neurosensory
- Muscular dystrophy, Duchenne-like ○
- Breast cancer BRCA 2
- Retinoblastoma △
- Osteosarcoma
- Wilson disease ○
- Propionicacidemia
- Xeroderma pigmentosum group G ○
- Clotting factor VII deficiency
- Clotting factor X deficiency

Chromosome 14
- Hypertrophic cardiomyopathy 1 △
- Glycogen storage VI (Hers)
- Nucleoside phosphorylase deficiency
- Galactosylceramide lipidosis
- Elliptocytosis (β-spectrin defect)
- Spherocytosis type 1 △
- α₁-antitrypsin deficiency ○
- Transcortin deficiency
- Porphyria variegata
- Usher syndrome type 1 ○
- Spinocerebellar ataxia 3

C. Gene loci for diseases in man (chromosomes 9-14)

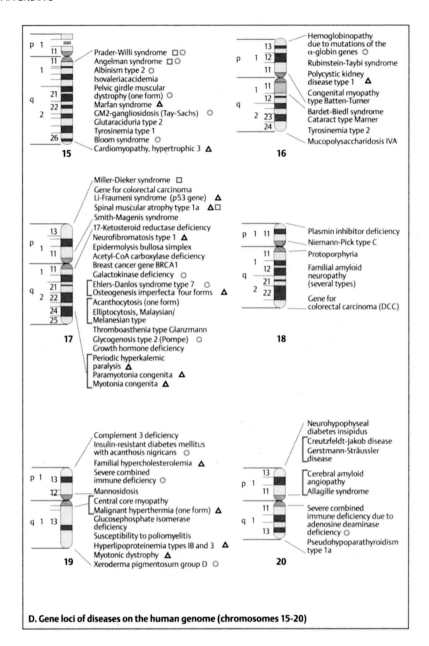

D. Gene loci of diseases on the human genome (chromosomes 15-20)

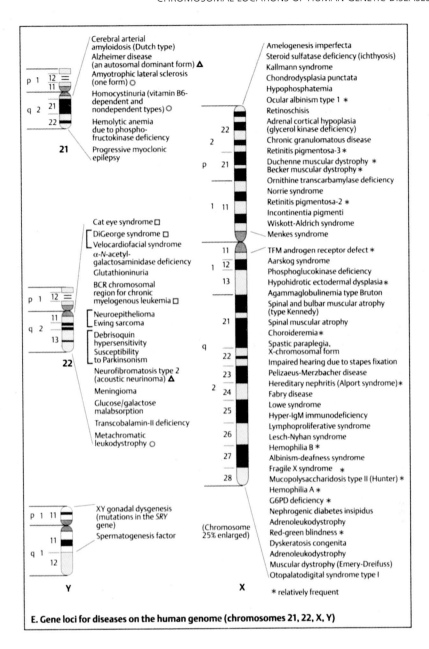

E. Gene loci for diseases on the human genome (chromosomes 21, 22, X, Y)

Figure Credits

Chapter 1

Figure 1-1B: From Swanson TA, Kim SI, Glucksman MJ. *BRS Biochemistry and Molecular Biology*. 4th ed. Baltimore: Lippincott Williams & Wilkins, 2007:341, fig. 21-2.

Chapter 2

Figure 2-1: From Dudek RW. *BRS Genetics*. 1st ed. Baltimore: Lippincott Williams & Wilkins, 2010:22, fig. 3-1.

Figure 2-3: From Dudek RW. *BRS Genetics*. 1st ed. Baltimore: Lippincott Williams & Wilkins, 2010:117, fig. 11-6A, B.

Figure 2-4: From Dudek RW. *BRS Genetics*. 1st ed. Baltimore: Lippincott Williams & Wilkins, 117, fig. 11-6C, E.

Chapter 6

Figure 6-1: From Dudek RW. *HY Cell and Molecular Biology*. 1st ed. Baltimore: Lippincott Williams & Wilkins, 1999:37, fig. 7-1.

Original source: Redrawn from Alberts B, Bray D, Johnson A, et al. *Essential Cell Biology*. New York: Garland Science, 1998: 264.

Figure 6-2: Dudek RW. *HY Cell and Molecular Biology*. 1st ed. Baltimore: Lippincott Williams & Wilkins, 1999:45, fig. 8-3.

Original source: Reproduced with permission from Alberts B, Bray D, Johnson A, et al. *Essential Cell Biology*. New York: Garland Science, 1998:230.

Chapter 7

Figure 7-2A: From Dudek RW. *HY Cell and Molecular Biology*. 1st ed. Baltimore: Lippincott Williams & Wilkins, 1999:38, fig. 7-2.

Original source: From Alberts B, Bray D, Johnson A, et al. *Essential Cell Biology*. New York: Garland Science, 1998:268.

Figures 7-2 to 7-5: From Dudek RW. *HY Cell and Molecular Biology*. 1st ed. Baltimore: Lippincott Williams & Wilkins, 1999:39, fig. 7-3.

Chapter 9

Figure 9-1: From Dudek RW. *HY Genetics*. 1st ed. Lippincott Williams & Wilkins, 2010:178, fig. 16-3.

Figure 9-2: From Dudek RW. *HY Genetics*. 1st ed. Lippincott Williams & Wilkins, 2010:179, fig. 16-4.

Figure 9-3: From Dudek RW. *HY Genetics*. 1st ed., Lippincott Williams & Wilkins, 2010:180, fig. 16-5.

Figure 9-4: From Dudek RW. *BRS Genetics*. 1st ed., Lippincott Williams & Wilkins, 2010:181, fig. 16-6A, B.

Figure 9-5: From Dudek RW. *BRS Genetics*. 1st ed. Lippincott Williams & Wilkins, 2010:181, fig. 16-6C.

Figure 9-6: From Dudek RW. *BRS Genetics*. 1st ed. Lippincott Williams & Wilkins, 2010:181, fig. 16-6E, F.

Figure 9-7: From Dudek RW. *BRS Genetics*. 1st ed. Lippincott Williams & Wilkins, 2010:181, fig. 16-6D.

Chapter 10

Table 10-1: From Dudek RW. *HY Cell and Molecular Biology*. 2nd ed. Lippincott Williams & Wilkins, 2007:128.

Figure 10-1: From Dudek RW. *BRS Genetics*. 1st ed. Baltimore: Lippincott Williams & Wilkins, 2010:172, fig. 16-2.

Chapter 11

Figures 11-1 to 11-4: From Dudek RW. *HY Cell and Molecular Biology*. 2nd ed. Lippincott Williams & Wilkins, 2007:131, fig. 16-1.

Chapter 12

Figure 12-9: From Dudek RW: HY Histopathology, 1st ed. Baltimore: Lippincott Williams and Wilkins, 2008:151, fig. 12-2.

Chapter 13

Figure 13-5: From Rubin R, Strayer DS. *Rubin's Pathology*. 5th ed. Baltimore: Lippincott Williams & Wilkins; 2008:1139, figs. 26-54 and 26-55A.

Figure 13-6 (top): From Brandt WE, Helms CA. *Fundamentals of Diagnostic Radiology*. 2nd ed. Baltimore: Lippincott Williams & Wilkins, 1999:993, fig. 42.24.

Figure 13-6 (bottom): From Damjanov I. *Histopathology: A Color Atlas and Textbook*. 1st ed. Baltimore: Lippincott Williams & Wilkins, 1996:176, plate 7.10, fig. 7-31A, B (inset).

Figure 13-7: From Rubin R, Strayer DS. *Rubin's Pathology*. 5th ed. Baltimore: Lippincott Williams & Wilkins, 2008:1212, fig. 28-69A.

Chapter 15

Figure 15-1: From McMillan JA, DeAngelis CD, Feigin RD, Warshaw JB. *Oski's Pediatrics: Principles and Practice*. 3rd ed. Baltimore: Lippincott Williams & Wilkins, 1999:2248, left side of page no figure number.

Figure 15-2: From McMillan JA, DeAngelis CD, Feigin RD, Warshaw JB. *Oski's Pediatrics: Principles and Practice*. 3rd ed. Baltimore: Lippincott Williams & Wilkins, 1999:2249, right side of page no figure number.

Figure 15-3: From McMillan JA, DeAngelis CD, Feigin RD, Warshaw JB. *Oski's Pediatrics: Principles and Practice*. 3rd ed. Baltimore: Lippincott Williams & Wilkins, 1999:2254, left side of page no figure number.

Figure 15-4: From McMillan JA, DeAngelis CD, Feigin RD, Warshaw JB. *Oski's Pediatrics: Principles and Practice*. 3rd ed. Baltimore: Lippincott Williams & Wilkins, 1999:2251, left side of page no figure number.

Index

Note: Italicized *f*'s and *t*'s refer to figures and tables

A

acute promyelocytic leukemia (APL), 53
adeno-associated virus vectors, 135
adenosine deaminase deficiency (ADA), 95, 126*f*, 128
adenoviruses, 135
agglutination, 92
alignment, 17
all-aneuploidy theory, 72
alternative internal promoters, 45
alternative promoters, 44–5
*Alu*1 enzyme, 100*f*, 101
amino acids, 138*f*
anaphase, 68
aneuploidy, 72
anticodon arm, 37
antigen-presenting cells, 80
antigens, 83
antisense RNA genes, 24, 44
AP1, 40
apoptosis, 71
arms, 7
ataxia-telangiectasia, 14–5
autoimmune disorders, 97–9
 organ-specific, 97–9
 systemic, 97

B

B lymphocytes, 89–93
 early immune response, 81
 hemopoietic stem cells, 81
 immature B cells, 81
 immunoglobulin diversity, 90
 immunoglobulin function, 92
 immunoglobulin properties, 90–2
 immunoglobulin structure, 89–90
 later immune response, 81–2
 mature B cells, 81
 pre-B cells, 81
bacterial artificial chromosomes (BACs), 109
Barr body, 45
base excision repair, 13
basophils, 78
Becker muscular dystrophy (DMD), 51
beta-thalassemia, 38
blood disorders, 97–8
BOR (branchio-oto-renal) syndrome, 131
branchio-oto-renal (BOR) syndrome, 131
BRCA1 hereditary breast cancer, 65
BRCA2 hereditary breast cancer, 65
breast cancer, 65

C

C banding, 6
cAMP response element binding protein, 40, 42

cancer, 71–3
 development of, 71–2
 progression of, 72–3
 accumulation of mutational events, 72–3
 chromosome instability, 72–3
 DNA repair, 72–3
 microsatellite instability, 72–3
 signal transduction pathways, 73–6
cancer stem cells, formation of, 72
CAP binding site, 47
caretaker tumor-suppressor genes, 61, 62*t*
catabolite activator protein (CAP), 46–7
CD8+ T lymphocytes, 126*f*, 127
Cdk-cyclin complexes, 68
cDNA library, 110*f*, 111
C/EBP protein, 41
cell cycle, 66–9
 control of, 68–9
 diagram of, 70*f*
 mitosis, 66–8
cell division, 17–9
central nervous system (CNS) disorders, 98–9
centromeres, 4
cerebral gigantism, 129
CHARGE association, 131
checkpoints, 68–9
Chediak-Higashi syndrome (CHS), 96
chemiluminescent substrate, 121
chemokines, 87
chimeric mice, 116*f*, 117
chromatin fiber, 3
chromosome 18, diagram of, 18*f*
chromosomes, 5–7
 banding, 5–6
 compaction, 4
 general features, 7
 instability, 72–3
 meiotic, 5
 mitotic, 5
 morphology, 7
 nomenclature, 7
 painting, 6
 replication, 9–16
 DNA damage, 12–3
 DNA repair, 13
 DNA replication machinery, 16*t*
 DNA topoisomerases, 11–2
 process, 9–11
 telomere, 12
 staining, 5–6
chronic myeloid leukemia (CML), 53
cis-acting DNA sequences, 39–40
classic gene family, 23
clonal selection theory, 89–99
cloning, 108*f*, 109–11, 112*f*
cloning vector, 109
close clustering, 23
Cockayne syndrome, 14
codon, third nucleotide of, 50
colinearity principle, 33

comparative genome hybridization (CGH), 6–7
complement activation, 92
compound cluster, 23
congenital thymic aplasia, 96
conservative substitutions, 50
conservative transposition, 27
core promoter sequence, 39
cosmid vectors, 109
creatine phosphokinase, 51
Cre-loxP recombination system, 117
crossover, 17
cyclin-dependent protein kinases (Cdks), 68
cyclins, 68–9
cytokines, 87–8
    activities, 88t
    chemokines, 87
    properties, 87
    receptors, 87
cytokinesis, 68
cytosine, deamination of, 13
cytotoxicity, 92

D

D arm, 37
deamination, 13
deletion polymorphism, 57
deoxyribonucleoside 5'-triphosphates, 10
deoxyribonucleoside triphosphates, 104f, 105
depurination, 13
diabetic embryopathy, 131
dideoxyribonucleoside triphosphates, 104f, 105
differential display PCR, 113
DiGeorge syndrome, 96, 126f, 127–8
diploid, 66
disjunction, 17–9
DNA, 1–8
    base composition, 8
    chemical environment, 8
    chemical modification of, 25
    denaturation, 8
    double helix, 2
    melting curve, 8
    noncoding, 25–8
        microsatellite DNA, 25–6
        minisatellite DNA, 25–6
        satellite DNA, 25
        transposons, 26–8
    polynucleotide chain, 2f
    supercoiling, 11
    topoisomerases, 11–2
DNA cloning, 108f, 109–11, 112f
DNA damage, 12–3
DNA polymerases, 11
DNA primase, 11
DNA repair, 13, 72–3
DNA sequencing, 104f, 105, 131
DNA-binding proteins, 41–3
    helix-loop-helix protein, 43
    homeodomain proteins, 41
    leucine zipper proteins, 42
    zinc finger proteins, 43
DNA-binding transcription factor, 132
downstream sequences, 33
Duchenne muscular dystrophy (DMD), 51
dwarfism, 41
dynamic mutations, 53–5
dystrophin, 51

E

early instability theory, 72
*Eco*R1 enzyme, 100f, 101
electrophoresis, 102f, 103
ELISA test, 122f, 123
encephalopathy, 32
endocytosis, receptor-mediated, 136

endogenous antigens, 83
    immune response to, 86–7
enhancer sequences, 39
enzyme-linked immunoabsorbent assay (ELISA) test, 122f, 123
eosinophil chemotactic factor, 79
eosinophils, 78
epigenetic control, 23, 25
episomes, 134, 135–6
euchromatin, 5, 10
ex vivo gene therapy, 134
exogenous antigens, 83
    early response to, 85
    late response to, 85–6
exons, 23
expression vector, 114f, 115
EYA1 protein, 131

F

familial adenomatous polyposis coli (FAPC), 64
flow cytometry, 126f, 127
fluorescence in situ hybridization (FISH), 6
FOS protein, 42
fragile X syndrome, 54
frameshift mutations, 51

G

G banding, 5–6
G$_0$ (gap) phase, 66
G$_1$ checkpoint, 66, 68
G$_1$ phase, 66
G$_2$ checkpoint, 66, 69
G$_2$ phase, 66
gain of function mutation, 55–6
gatekeeper tumor-suppressor genes, 60, 62t
gene expression, 39–48
    definition of, 115
    mechanisms of, 39–40, 41f, 44–6
        cis-acting DNA sequences, 39–40
        trans-acting proteins, 40
gene knockout, 116f, 117
gene regulatory proteins, 40
gene superfamily, 23
gene therapy, 133–6
    episomes, 134
    ex vivo, 134
    germ-line, 133
    host cell chromosomes, 134
    nonviral vectors, 135–6
        direct injection, 135
        liposomes, 135
        receptor-mediated endocytosis, 135
    somatic cell, 133
    viral vectors, 134–5
        adeno-associated, 135
        adenoviral, 135
        herpes simplex, 135
        lentivirus, 135
        oncoretroviral, 134
    in vivo, 134
genes
    cluster, 23
    dispersed, 23
    multiple clusters, 23
    truncated, 23
genetic code, 137t
genetic diseases, chromosomal locations of, 139–45
genetic recombination, 18f
    general recombination, 19
    site-specific, 19
genomic imprinting, 25
germ-line gene therapy, 133
growth factors, 60t
gyrases, 12

H

haploid, 66
helix-loop-helix protein, 43
hematopoietin, 87
hemophilia B, 115
hemopoietic stem cells, 81, 83
heparins, 79
hereditary cancer syndromes, 62–5
    BRCA1 and BRCA2 hereditary breast cancers, 65
    development of, 71
    familial adenomatous polyposis coli, 64
    Li-Fraumen syndrome, 63
    neurofibromatosis type 1, 63–4
    retinoblastoma, 62–3
hereditary nonpolyposis colorectal cancer (HNPCC), 15
herpes simplex viruses, 135
heterochromatin, 4, 10
*Hind*III enzyme, 100*f*, 101
histamine, 79
histiocytes, 80
histone methyltransferase, 129
histones, 3
    chemical modification of, 25
    positively charged, 121
homeobox sequence, 41
homeodomain proteins, 41
host cell chromosomes, 134
housekeeping genes, 39–48
housekeeping proteins, 39–48
hsp70, 40
human disease gene identification, 129–32
    chromosome abnormality, 129
    comparison of human and mouse maps, 131–2
    DNA sequencing, 131
    transcript mapping, 130
human Factor IX, 115
human Factor VIII, 109
human genetic diseases, chromosomal locations of, 139–45
human immunodeficiency virus (HIV)
    ELISA test, 122*f*, 123
    structure, 122*f*, 123
    Western blot test, 122*f*, 123
Huntington disease, 54–5
hypermutation, 82

I

IgA, 91–2
IgD, 91
IgE, 91
IgG, 91
IgM, 90–1
immune system, 77–99
    cell biology of, 77–88
    clonal selection theory, 89
    disorders of phagocytic function, 96–7
    molecular biology of, 89–99
    organ-specific autoimmune disorders, 97–9
    systemic autoimmune disorders, 97
immunoglobulin (IG), 89–92
    agglutination, 92
    complement activation, 92
    cytotoxicity, 92
    gene rearrangement, 90
    heavy chains, 89
    insertional diversity, 90
    junctional diversity, 90
    light chains, 89
    neutralization, 92
    opsonization, 92
    properties, 93
    somatic cell mutations, 90
in vivo gene therapy, 134
insertion polymorphism, 57
insulator sequences, 39
interleukin, 88*t*

internal gene fragments, 23
introns, 23, 50
inverse PCR, 113
isotype switching, 82

J

JUN protein, 42

K

karyotype chaos, 71
Kearns-Sayre syndrome (KS), 31–2

L

lac operon, 46–7
lactic acidosis, 32
Leber's hereditary optic neuropathy (LHON), 31–2
lentiviruses, 135
leucine zipper proteins, 42
leukotrienes, 79
Li-Fraumen syndrome (LFS), 63
ligase chain reaction (LCR), 124*f*, 125
liposomes, 135
long interspersed nuclear elements (LINEs), 26
long terminal repeat transposons, 26
loss of function mutation, 55

M

macrophages, 80
Martin-Bell syndrome, 54
mast cells, 78–9
maternal RNA, 45–6
meiosis, 19–20
    vs. mitosis, 21*t*
meiosis I, 17–9
    alignment, 17
    cell division, 17–9
    crossover, 17
    disjunction, 17–9
    synapsis, 17
meiotic chromosomes, 5
Mep-1, 40
metaphase, 5, 68
micro RNA (miRNA) genes, 24, 44
microsatellite DNA, 25–6
microsatellite DNA polymorphism, 57
microsatellite instability, 72–3
Miller syndrome, 131
minisatellite DNA, 25–6
minisatellite DNA polymorphism, 57
mismatch repair, 13
missense mutations, 50
mitochondrial diseases, 31–2
mitochondrial genome, 29–32
    general features, 29
    location of mtDNA genes and gene products, 30*f*
    protein-coding genes, 29, 30*t*
    RNA-coding genes, 29, 30*t*
mitochondrial myopathy, encephalopathy, lactic acidosis, and stroke-like episodes syndrome (MELAS), 32
mitochondrial proteins, 31
mitosis, 66–8
    vs. meiosis, 21*t*
mitotic chromosomes, 5
modified standard theory of cancer, 71
molecular biology techniques, 100–28
    DNA cloning, 108*f*, 109–11, 112*f*
    DNA sequencing, 104*f*, 105
    polymerase chain reaction, 113–28
    restriction enzymes, 100–4
monocytes, 79–80
multiple myeloma, 97–8
multiple sclerosis, 98–9

mutagenesis, 116f, 117
mutations, 49–57
    base substitutions, 49
    cancer progression and, 72–3
    gain of function, 55–6
    general features, 49
    loss of function, 55
    non-silent (nonsynonymous) mutations, 50–4
        dynamic mutations, 53–5
        frameshift mutations, 51
        missense mutations, 50
        nonsense mutations, 50
        RNA splicing mutations, 52
        translocation mutations, 52–3
        transposon mutations, 52
    point, 58
    silent (synonymous), 49–50
    translocation, 58–9
myasthenia gravis, 99
MYC protein, 42
myeloperoxidase deficiency (MPO), 96
myoclonic epilepsy with ragged red fibers syndrome
        (MERRF), 31
MyoD protein, 42

N

Nager syndrome, 131
natural killer CD16$^+$ cells, 81
negative selection, 83
negative supercoiling, 11
neurofibromatosis type 1, 63–4
neutralization, 92
neutrophils, 77
nitrogenous bases, 1
noncoding DNA, 25–8. *See also* DNA
    microsatellite DNA, 25–6
    minisatellite DNA, 25–6
    satellite DNA, 25
    transposons, 26–8
nonconservative substitutions, 50
nonsense mutations, 50
Northern blot, 118f, 119
NSD1 protein, 129
nuclear genome, 22–8
    epigenetic control, 25
    general features, 22–3
    noncoding DNA, 25–8
    protein-coding genes, 23–4
nucleic acids, 1
nucleosides, 1
nucleosome, 3
nucleotide excision repair, 13

O

oncogenes. *See also* proto-oncogenes
    alteration of proto-oncogenes to, 58–9
    definition of, 58
oncogenesis, 71–2
    all-aneuploidy theory, 72
    early instability theory, 72
    formation of cancer stem cells, 72
    modified standard theory, 71
    standard theory, 71
oncoretroviruses, 134
opsonization, 92
organ-specific autoimmune disorders, 97–9

P

P1 artificial chromosomes (P1 artificial chromosomes), 109
palindromes, 100f, 101
PAX3 gene, 131–2
petit arms, 7
Philadelphia chromosome, 58
phosphates, 1

pituitary dwarfism, 41
plasmid vector, 109
point mutation, 58
polymerase chain reaction (PCR), 113–28
    chimeric mice, 116f
    differential display, 113
    ELISA test, 122f, 123
    expression vector, 114f, 115
    flow cytometry, 126f
    gene knockout, 116f, 117
    inverse, 113
    ligase chain reaction, 124f, 125
    mutagenesis, 116f, 117
    Northern blot, 118f, 119
    real-time, 113
    reverse transcription, 113
    viral detection, 112f, 113
    Western blot, 120f, 121
polymorphisms, 49
positive selection, 83
positive supercoiling, 11
prenatal testing, 106f, 107
processed pseudogenes, 23
prometaphase, 5, 66
prophase, 66
protein synthesis, 33–8
    general features, 33
    processing RNA transcript into mRNA, 34–5
    transcription, 33–4
    translation, 35–7
protein-coding genes, 23–4
proto-oncogene, 58–60
proto-oncogenes
    alteration to oncogene, 58–9
    amplification, 58
    definition of, 58
    growth factors, 60t
    point mutation, 58
    RAS, 59
    receptors, 60t
    signal transducers, 60t
    transcription factors, 60t
    translocation, 58
proximal promoter region sequence, 39
pseudogenes, 23–4
purines, 1
pyrimidine, 1

Q

Q banding, 6
queue arm, 7

R

R banding, 6
RAS gene, 59
RB1 gene, 61
real-time PCR, 113
receptors, 60t
recombinant plasmid, 109
regulatory RNA genes, 24
repetitive DNA sequences, 23
replication, 9–11
    bubble, 9, 10f
    fork, 10f, 11
    origins, 9
    prokaryotic DNA, 11
response element sequences, 40
restriction enzymes (REs), 100–4
retinoblastoma, 61, 62–3
retrogenes, 23
retrotransposition, 27
reverse gyrase, 12
reverse transcription PCR, 113
rheumatoid arthritis, 97
ribosomal RNA (rRNA) genes, 24
riboswitch genes, 24

riboswitch RNA, 44
RNA capping, 34
RNA polyadenylation, 34
RNA polymerases, 33
RNA splicing, 35, 45
RNA splicing mutations, 52
RNA-binding proteins, 45
RNA-coding genes, 23, 24
Robertsonian translocation, 52–3

S

S (synthesis) phase, 66
satellite DNA, 25
serum response factor, 40
severe combined immune deficiency (SCID), 95
short interspersed nuclear elements (SINEs), 26
sickle cell anemia, 100*f*, 101, 106*f*, 107
signal transducers, 60*t*
signal transduction pathways, 73–6
    mitogen-activated protein kinase, 74*f*
    phosphatidylinositol 3-kinase/PTEN/AKT, 76*f*
    transforming growth factor, 75*f*
silencer sequences, 39
silent (synonymous) mutations, 49–50
simple sequence repeat (SSR) polymorphism, 57
single nucleotide polymorphisms, 49
site-specific recombination, 19
small interfering (siRNA) genes, 24, 44
small nuclear (snRNA) genes, 24
small nucleolar (snoRNA) genes, 24
somatic cell gene therapy, 133
Sotos syndrome, 129
Southern blotting, 106*f*, 107
spacer DNA, 49
Splotch (Sp) mutant, 132
sporadic cancers, 71
standard theory of cancer, 71
stat-1, 40
stem cells, 72
    adult, 83
    embryonic, 83
    hemopoietic, 83
steroid hormone receptor, 40
subbands, 7
subregions, 7
sub-subbands, 7
sugars, 1
supercoiling, 11
synapsis, 17
systemic autoimmune disorders, 97
systemic lupus erythematosus (SLE), 37–8

T

TΨC arm, 37
T banding, 6
T cells, 83
T lymphocytes, 94–5
    endogenous antigens, 83
    exogenous antigens, 83
    hemopoietic stem cells, 83
    immature T cells, 83
    mature T cells, 83
    negative selection, 83
    positive selection, 83
    T-cell receptor diversity, 94–5
    T-cell receptor structure, 94
telomere, 12
telophase, 68
topoisomerases, 11–2
Towne-Brocks syndrome, 131
TP53 gene, 61–2
trans-acting proteins, 40
transcript mapping, 130

transcription, 33–4
transcription factors, 40, 60*t*
transfer RNA (tRNA) genes, 37
transitions, 49
translation, 35–7
translocation mutations, 52–3, 58–9
transposons, 26–8
    conservative transposition, 27
    DNA, 26
    genetic variability and, 27–8
    long interspersed nuclear elements, 26
    long terminal repeat, 26
    mechanisms of, 26–7
    mutations, 52
    retrotransposition, 27
    short interspersed nuclear elements, 26
transversions, 49
Treacher-Collins Franceschetti syndrome, 130
trp operon, 47–8
truncated genes, 23
tryptophan, 47–8
tumor necrosis factor, 88*t*
tumor-suppressor genes, 60–2
    caretaker, 61, 62*t*
    gatekeeper, 60, 62*t*
    RB1, 61
    TP53, 61–2
22q11.12 deletion syndrome, 95–6

U

unequal crossover, 56
unequal sister chromatid exchange (UESCE), 57
unprocessed pseudogenes, 23
upstream sequences, 33
uracil, deamination of cytosine to, 13

V

variable number tandem repeat (VNTR) polymorphisms, 56–7
    large-scale, 57
    replication slippage in, 57
    simple, 57
    unequal crossover in, 56
    unequal sister chromatid exchange in, 57
viral vectors, 134–5
    adeno-associated, 135
    adenoviral, 135
    herpes simplex, 135
    lentivirus, 135
    oncoretroviral, 134
von Recklinghausen disease, 63–4

W

Waardenburg syndrome type 1, 131–2
Warthin-Lynch syndrome, 14–5
Western blot, 120*f*, 121, 122*f*, 123

X

X chromosome inactivation, 45
xeroderma pigmentosum, 14
x-linked infantile agammaglobulinemia (XLA), 95, 126*f*, 127

Y

yeast artificial chromosomes (YACs), 109

Z

zinc finger proteins, 43